MOTIV

AND FIT

STRATEGIES TO CREATE A TENACIOUS MINDSET AND ASTONISHING BODY AT ANY AGE!

MOTIVATED AND FIT

STRATEGIES TO CREATE A TENACIOUS MINDSET AND ASTONISHING BODY AT ANY AGE!

JOEL LUCKY

GET WRITE PUBLISHING

Motivated and Fit: Strategies to Create a Tenacious Mindset and Astonishing Body at Any Age

Copyright © 2019 by Joel Lucky

ISBN: 978-1-7337020-6-5

Cover Design: USEntarprise

Get Write Publishing
2770 Main Street – Suite 147
Frisco, TX 75033

DEDICATION

Much love to my beautiful wife Julie, who is always my rock and without whose help this book would not exist. I adore you and appreciate you in a way that words aren't sufficient to express.

The ultimate in gratitude to my incredibly encouraging mom, Joan, and my uplifting dad, Joe. The two of you have always instilled in me that I could do anything. I would not be where I am today without you.

Special thanks to Karen Shaw of Hello World Photography for the cover shot of *Motivated and Fit*.

TABLE OF CONTENTS

SECTION 2: THE BODY

WHO I AM

Since the age of 12, I have had a strong desire to be muscular and fit. Now at age 54, I am just as fascinated with physical development as I have ever been. My formal education includes attaining certifications from the National Academy of Sports Medicine and multiple certifications from the Cooper Institute in Dallas, Texas. I also have a B.S. in Occupational Therapy from the University of Louisiana at Monroe and a M.S. degree from the University of Southern Mississippi.

However, the above credentials are not the reason you might consider reading what I have to say. An individual preaching the fitness gospel must be able to walk his talk. If your author does not really work out and train intensely with respectable weights on a regular basis, as well as look the part, they are probably not the information source you are looking for. An academic theorizer who appears as though he or she couldn't punch their way out of a wet paper bag can't really be a credible instructor. Neither is the author who owes a large part of his/her physique development to the use of illegal performance enhancing drugs.

The photo on the cover of this book was taken just five weeks shy of my 54th birthday. No airbrushing of the photo or any other tomfoolery was used the day this was taken. This is not to impress you, but to impress upon you that your author has both the knowledge of exercise science and **more importantly**, real-world exercise experience. I have put my money where my mouth is by multiple top three finishes and first place wins in several body building competitions (more on that later). I have also achieved the coveted natural powerlifting benchmarks of 300+ pounds, 400+ pounds, and 500+ pounds in the bench press, squat, and deadlift respectively.

To steroid assisted athletes, these accomplishments are no big deal. To the genetically typical and/or non-PED using trainee, these accomplishments are quite respectable. And if I have been able to do this, YOU can achieve physical prowess that is just as impressive. I am nothing special. I am merely an individual who has been motivated as heck that has both the formal education and practical hands-on experience in the area of building the body.

I have a successful personal training background dating back to the early 1990s and have spent literally thousands of hours helping others become their physical best. A blueprint for YOU to become YOUR physical best will be provided in the following text!

ABOUT THIS BOOK

Going way back to when I was a teenager, I have always had an intense desire to motivate and inspire people to achieve their dreams—especially those who would consider themselves as being the underdog compared to their peers; whether due to either their own self-limiting beliefs or how they have allowed outside influences make them feel. I am a true believer that everyone has the seeds of greatness within them.

Since the mid-1980s, I have had a passion for learning the keys to both personal and physical development. I have spent literally thousands of hours studying personal development gurus such as Jonathan Parker and Anthony Robbins. This was done to create a tenacious mindset that would equip me to face any challenge that might come my way in life. On the physical development front, much time was spent learning how old school natural bodybuilders and powerlifters such as Reg Park and Brooks Kubik built their awe-inspiring strength and physiques. For over three decades, I have used my own mind and body as a laboratory to acquire refined proficiency in these areas.

During the summer of 2018, I decided it was finally time for me to share what I learned with the world. As a 54-year-old with a wife, two teenage boys, and a job, I wanted to show everyone how to be their personal best, **despite busy life circumstances and age!**

THE CHALLENGE

Our world is becoming more fast paced than ever before. People do not have a lot of time to even read something brief like a 10-page chapter. Those that do have the time have been conditioned by external forces to not invest time in reading long books. People now want their information to be given to them quickly, succinctly, and efficiently. No excessive wordiness, no fluff.

Would writing a book the conventional way be the best vehicle to deliver the information that I wanted to provide my readers? With the advent of social media and its constant evolution over the years, the majority of individuals have a preference towards taking in new information in bite-sized pieces. Thus, I surmised that a book written with very brief chapters covering a multitude of personal development and fitness concepts would fit the bill of today's reader. This is what I have done with this book.

Motivated and Fit was born through an idea that I decided to make part of my daily routine on June 1, 2018. Each morning, I would get up, drink my favorite caffeine/amino acid supplement, and get my iPad ready. The goal was to pick a topic, thought, or story that would be helpful to anyone of any age in the areas of the mind and body. And write. Just write. The only criteria being that it would be about methods that have been proven to work and would be of benefit to you, the reader. The best of these morning compositions make up the contents of this book. *Motivated and Fit* is a compilation of small chapters focused on building your will, building motivation to achieve your hopes and dreams, creating fitness, and inspirational stories of unlikely high-achievers who defied the odds.

The first part of the book is about how to motivate yourself for victory and utilize strategies for success. You will learn a game plan of forging a mindset that enables you to avoid psychological landmines; the snares of life that often result in defeat. I am a big proponent of helping others help themselves. Thus, much of the early chapters teach a concept or tell a story for you to ponder upon. This will be followed by a section for you to write down how what you have just read can be applied to your life. The mindset portion of *Motivated and Fit* has a bit of a workbook feel. Whether your goal is success in the boardroom or on the beach, this book has something for everyone!

The second part of the book is about becoming the fittest you possible! The *Motivated and Fit* Weight Training System is a time tested, proven way to build your best physique ever. It is based on basic exercises, consistency, and simplicity. Conventional training methods and ideology are not promoted in this text. The reason for this is that conventional methods simply do not work for the majority of people. Only nuts and bolts information will be provided.

Glossy muscle photos and monotonous exercise explanations can be found all over the internet and social media, as well as in hundreds of exercise encyclopedias. Programming to build the body of your dreams in the most efficient manner possible is what this book is all about. Real world nutrition and cardiovascular training information are explained in a simple, easy to understand manner. You will learn that becoming fit is not rocket science!

No matter how much or how little you know about the art and science of building muscle and becoming fit, there is something for everyone in this book. Even for those with little interest in physical goals, there is a treasure trove of information in the following pages on how to harness the power of the mind. *Motivated and Fit* will challenge you to utilize your God-given greatness; a greatness that you will learn resides inside of you and is yearning to reveal itself to the world! This book is not the last word on strength and health nor is it an exhaustive manual that covers every possible fitness subject. However, it is a composition that is filled with information that will greatly help just about any fitness enthusiast. I hope you enjoy the information in the upcoming chapters as much as I have enjoyed writing it for YOU!

Chapter 1

CAJUN COUNTRY

My childhood and teenage years were for the most part quite pleasant. Luling, Louisiana was a very friendly town made up predominantly of charming Acadian-French descendants. I was blessed to have a group of caring, encouraging friends. On the other hand, I also had my share of dealing with discouraging, hateful naysayers. At a young age in this environment, I learned the following: people can be negative. Many like to gain power over others by using words that are intended to hurt and discourage. "You can't do it." "You don't have what it takes." "You're not good enough." If you are ever told anything like this, don't take the bait. You can choose to fall for ill-intentioned statements and let it deflate your balloon, or you can use it to light a fire under you and resolve to prove them wrong.

During my teenage years, this was something I faced from a couple of young guys that I will call Ted and Trey (names have been changed to protect the not-so-innocent). They were both in the class ahead of me at Hahnville High School, nestled in the heart of Cajun country, about 20 miles west of New Orleans. Both boys were more physically mature and muscular than I was. In my junior year of high school (1982), I was working out hard, but my body was just not ready hormonally to blossom with muscle. I was a classic late bloomer. It clearly wasn't my time.

1

One day in the gym, Trey and Ted spotted me and decided to use me for target practice. Trey said "Lucky, you are just wasting your time, bruh." (In south Louisiana, "bruh" is "bro" to the rest of the world). You work out hard but don't have the right kind of body to build any muscle. You just don't have what it takes to get big." Ted smugly looked at me with a condescending smirk and vigorously nodded his head in agreement. I replied to Trey's verbal assault with "Trey, not only am I going to get big, one day I'm going to enter a bodybuilding contest and win." Both of them laughed at me quite mockingly, calling over some buddies to let them know what I said in an effort to pile on the humiliation. I could have allowed this to discourage me. Instead, I resolved at this time to use such situations moving forward as fuel. This fuel was just what I needed to help drive me to what I knew would be my destiny in many areas.

Fast forward to August of 1991. A lot had happened since 1982. I was no longer the shy, skinny, awkward teenager that I was in high school. I had attained a college degree and had been out in the real world for several years. I was an account manager at a hotel in Savannah, Georgia. In the spring of 1991, victory was finally mine; I made a reality of the of proclamation I had made nine years ago to Trey and Ted by winning two bodybuilding competitions! (One more than what I confidently predicted in 1982).

Later that summer, I returned to my hometown to visit my parents. The day after I arrived, I made a trip down to one of the local gyms where my bodybuilding journey began. This was the same club where Trey and

Ted mocked me when I revealed my dream to them. I began my workout, and had the pleasure of running into a couple of people who I knew from high school. They were so kind and complimentary about what I had done with my physique! I'm not going to lie; it really felt good to be praised in the same building where I was once scorned and ridiculed. What was said to me by Trey and Ted entered my mind for the first time in a quite a while. However, it was a memory that now made me feel good inside. I suddenly recalled in that moment that I backed up what I said to them in spades.

Just when I thought it couldn't get much better, guess who walked in through the door just a few minutes later? It was Ted! I recognized his wide shoulders, thick chest, and curly black hair immediately. Ted gazed across the small gym in my direction. His eyes widened. His jaw literally dropped open. After standing there for a few seconds in stunned silence, Ted quickly walked across the gym floor towards me. I received an extended hand and a pleased look of resignation from him that expressed, "I remember what we told you and we were obviously wrong." As I grasped his enthusiastic handshake, Ted simply asked with true humbleness and sincerity, "Ok Joel, tell me what shows you have won!" I was slightly tempted to remind Ted of what he and Trey had stated to me so many years ago. I easily passed on that opportunity. In his own way, he admitted that he had to eat crow on what was said and was fine with doing so. I got the feeling he was trying to say "I'm sorry" without coming right out and saying it. This was good enough for me. I replied with something like "Well, I haven't won Mr. America or anything, but I did win a couple of smaller shows this past spring in Georgia." As a side note, Trey also ended up eating his words a few months earlier in a much more humbling fashion. But that is another story for another time.

To reiterate the point of the story: Believe in yourself even when no one else thinks you have a prayer. People will laugh at you, and people will pull against you. People will attempt to put doubt in your mind about what you can accomplish. You must have a dogged determination to press upward and onward despite the words of the naysayers. Proclaim your goals and dreams, make a plan, work your plan, envision victory, and make whatever you desire a reality. Make a promise to yourself that you will attain your dream no matter what!

SELF-MOTIVATIONAL MOMENT

I promise myself that I will attain my dream of:

_____

_____

_____

_____

Signature:

_____

Date:

_____

> "The first step toward success is taken when you refuse to be a captive of the environment in which you first find yourself."
> -Mark Caine

Chapter 2

JOIN THE 100% CLUB

As I was preparing for my first bodybuilding win back in the spring of 1991, a constant refrain from one of my youth football coaches kept running through my head: "Guys, you are going to play like you practice!" With this in mind, I gave 100% to all aspects of my contest preparation. Painstaking detail was given to my weight training program, nutrition plan, and posing. This was true even in my mental preparation. I would close my eyes and visualize standing atop the victory platform, holding my 1st place trophy high above my head. In a phone conversation with my brother the morning of the contest, I told him "Stafford, I don't know who's going to show up today, but I don't see anyone beating me." All out preparedness instills legitimate confidence.

The massive action that was given preparing for this contest resulted in victory! I have since carried the lesson I learned on giving 100% to all aspects of life since that time. We were all created to be, do, and achieve absolute excellence. However, excellence cannot be achieved without giving it everything you've got. All that you do paints a portrait as to the person that you are. Create a lifetime of masterpieces! To achieve this level of success, the actions taken to attain the desired result must not be half-hearted. Half-hearted effort equals half-hearted results.

Consistently give 100% to the things that are important for you to achieve. Roadblocks and obstacles will present themselves. You MUST navigate around these and quickly get back on course. Let nothing stop you. Remain steadfast in your efforts toward seizing the prize. As legendary distance runner Steve Prefontane once said, "To give less than 100% is to sacrifice the gift." Few people are willing to do what it takes to become a member of the 100% Club! Resolve today to be part of this winning group of individuals!

What areas of my life need 100% effort?

_____

_____

_____

_____

_____

> "We all have dreams. In order to make dreams come into reality, it takes an awful amount of determination, dedication, self-discipline, and effort."
>
> -Jesse Owens

8

Chapter 3

ROLE MODELING HIGH ACHIEVERS AND TAKING MASSIVE ACTION FOR SUCCESS

Tony Robbins presented an idea many years ago that has always stuck with me. Tony stated a simple thought about how to be successful in any area of life. Breaking it down, the basic message was:

1. Find someone who is successful in an area where you desire success.

2. Study what they did to become successful in that particular area.

3. Take massive action and do the same things that the high achiever did and get the same results.

Back in the early 1990s, I was not yet satisfied with my level of strength and size. I looked more like a fitness model than a bodybuilder. While I was strong compared to the layman, my strength was sub-par compared to some of the beasts I would watch train at the gym.

Fortunately, I purchased a subscription to an obscure magazine called *Hardgainer*. It was a publication dedicated to lifters that were drug-free and genetically typical. The training methodologies in *Hardgainer* were a far cry from what were in other muscle magazines at the time. Within these pages I found an author whose articles resonated with me. His name—Brooks Kubik.

Brooks Kubik was a veritable Hercules. He was drug-free and had a massive, dense physique. Brooks was a national bench press champion and was able to lift weights that would make many PED enhanced lifters envious. It was obvious to me that this was the combination of mass and strength that I wished to emulate. Studying the way Brooks trained began to radically alter the way I went about my business in the gym. I used Brooks' routines and methods, doing what he did to achieve his impressive results.

Massive action was taken in the gym! I trained like a demon in this new manner and utilized a training journal as a progress barometer. Over the next two years, I was able to put on 20 solid pounds of muscle with virtually no change in body fat levels. I surpassed the 300/400/500 poundage goals which I set for myself in the bench press, squat, and deadlift respectively. Imitating a high achiever like Brooks Kubik was the game plan that I put into play that yielded results which were previously unattainable.

People often try to reinvent the wheel when attempting to reach challenging goals. Why? If you have a goal in the area of personal development, there are high-achievers like Zig Ziglar, Anthony Robbins, and Billy Cox who have a ready-made game plan for you. Do you have a goal to improve as a natural powerlifter/weightlifter/bodybuilder? Iron men like Brooks Kubik and John Hansen have all of the information you will ever need to become your very best. Don't overthink the plans to reach your goals. Thinking about how to do something too much can actually delay you from taking the first step required to achieve results. Just find a high-achiever that has accomplished what you want to accomplish. Resolve to implement the tools and strategies that they utilized for success. MASSIVE ACTION is what is needed on your part! A template is useless without good old-fashioned hard work. Work daily towards the dreams and desires of your heart and separate yourself from the rest by imitating the best!

What high achiever do I need to role model?

_____

_____

_____

What massive action do I need to take?

_____

_____

_____

Infuse your life with action. Don't wait for it to happen. And whatever your beliefs, honor your creator, not by passively waiting for grace to come down from upon high, but by doing what you can to make grace happen... yourself, right now, right down here on Earth.

-Bradley Whitford

Chapter 4

DONT LET YOUR AGE GET IN YOUR HEAD

I am currently 54 years of age. Aches and pains are now a more common occurrence than in my younger years. My testosterone levels are not as high as they were in the 1980's, but you can't feel as though you are being defeated by Father Time.

You have to do the best you can with what you've got. You have to study the most recent findings in exercise science, nutrition, and supplementation. Find ways to rest, sleep, and recover better. Come on now! You can do it!

I have knuckled down the last two years to a new level and can honestly say that I'm physically superior now at age 54 to the version of myself at age 49! If I can do it, you can too! Yes, age has its challenges, but know that you can still make progress from where you are today if you don't let your age get in your head!

We sometimes become fearful to try new methods and ideas as we age. However, new approaches are often required in order to move forward as the clock ticks toward the second act of our lives. Research ways to beat the clock. Commit to being the best you that you can be DESPITE your age!

What are some areas I can study
to beat the clock?

_____

_____

_____

_____

_____

_____

_____

_____

"There is a fountain of youth: it is your mind, your talents, the creativity you bring to your life and the lives of the people you love. When you tap into this source, you will have truly defeated age."

-Sophia Loren

Chapter 5

HOW TO HAVE A POSITIVE MINDSET AT ANY AGE

Acquiring a positive mindset is something that both the old and young can develop in order to have a more fulfilling life. Benefits abound for those who CHOOSE to have a positive mindset. And, yes, whether you know it or not, having either a positive or negative mindset is a decision.

Those who think negatively are rarely happy, and the people that we interact with are greatly affected. Negative people will be avoided like a plague by all but a handful of people. A number of scientific studies have revealed that a positive mindset is directly related to having a more happy, successful, and profitable life. A positive mindset and resulting happiness and attraction from others is there for the taking. It requires just a little bit of effort. It is a relatively uncomplicated process whether you are age 12 or 72.

A few small adjustments to daily life can greatly enhance our mindset and make us and everyone we interact with much happier. Like an old TV commercial once said, "It is so simple even a caveman can do it."

Here is a list for developing a positive mindset:

Write Down 3 Things
You Are Grateful for Each Morning

Make a journal of the things you are grateful for. This will start your day on a positive note. The act of writing will reinforce the feeling of gratitude in your subconscious mind. Feelings of gratitude will greatly increase your joy and help insulate you from the negative effects of stress, anxiety, negativity, and depression. Starting each day feeling thankful can help balance out that negative experience we might have at work later on or an argument with a loved one.

Change How You View Your Challenges

No matter how we try, there are not many things in our lives that we have complete control over. You must not allow things that are beyond your control dishearten you. Encountering a roadblock does not mean you have to stop your car in the middle of the road. It means you have to take a detour and find your way back to the road you were traveling. View challenges as an opportunity for growth and adventure. Overcoming obstacles can be very gratifying and can provide a feeling of victory. Some of my most valued achievements were born of what most people would frame as disasters. I know it sounds corny and cliché, but "A setback is a set up for a comeback." And the feeling of making a comeback can be absolutely glorious! Just ask 2019 Masters Champion Tiger Woods!

Choose Your Words Carefully
When Describing Your Life

Words have power. Your mind will listen to your words and will subconsciously act to make these words reality, whether positive or negative. If you verbalize that your life is overwhelming, chaotic, or boring, these words will result in negative effects in your mind and body. Replacing these negative words with ones like involved, lively, and familiar will allow you to see your challenges in a more positive way. This will allow challenges to be met with positivity and more ability to overcome them.

Use Deep Breathing and Visualization
Each Morning

Upon awakening, think about one thing that you will do today that will make you smile. Lie flat on your back and close your eyes, taking in 10 deep breaths. Focus all of your attention on breathing in air through your nose and out through your mouth for 3 seconds each way. Clench and release your hands on each breathing cycle. Focus only on relaxing, breathing, and listening to yourself as you think of the thing that will make you smile. It could be petting your cat, going shopping with a friend, or watching a football game. This will help you establish a positive state of mind and a calmness to be able to handle the challenges of the day. It does not matter if you are a teenager navigating the turbulent waters of adolescence or a senior who is in their golden years of retirement. These strategies for facing challenges work for everyone. Put them into play immediately and watch the positive effects that they will have on your life.

CHAPTER NOTES

_____

_____

_____

_____

_____

_____

_____

_____

"Never underestimate the power you have to take your life in a new direction."

-Germany Kent

Chapter 6

EXCUSES... EXCUSES

We can always find an excuse for failure.
"I'm not smart."
"I don't have good genetics."
"I'm not pretty enough."
"I'm too old."
"I just can't get the right breaks."

The list goes on and on. Not taking personal responsibility for your own failure is a road to nowhere. It is easy to place the blame on other people and factors. Most of us have much more power inside of us than we ever come close to utilizing. It is up to **you** to make a plan as to how and why you will succeed rather than succumbing to your doubts and fears.

What are the excuses that I need to stop using?

_____

_____

_____

_____

"Never make excuses. Your friends don't need them and your foes won't believe them."

-John Wooden

Chapter 7

HOW TO ELIMINATE NEGATIVE THINKING

Many of us limit our potential by negative internal dialogue. Negative thoughts or images that continually saturate our mind will yield negative results toward accomplishing your goals. The next time you have a negative thought or image entering your mind, do the following: Close your eyes, take a deep breath, and let it out slowly. Imagine you're looking at a huge movie screen that is grey in color. Visualize a written list on the screen with negative beliefs such as:

- I am not talented.
- I am unattractive.
- I am not confident.

Then see the following words flash in rapid succession across the screen over the top of the negative statements:

- STOP
- DELETE
- CANCEL

Now see the words flash across the screen again, but this time repeat aloud what you are reading with pure emotion! Say aloud: STOP! DELETE! CANCEL!

Feel the positive rush through your body as you repeat this several times! Know that you're wiping out negative thoughts and negative self-talk patterns! With positive emotion, repeat positive statements such as:

"I AM SUCCESSFUL AT ALL I DO!"
"I EXUDE AND RADIATE CONFIDENCE!"
"EVERYTHING TURNS OUT RIGHT FOR ME!"

Visualize these positive statements on the screen in shiny gold letters. This will help program you to replace negative ramblings in your mind with positive feelings and statements. Resolve today to start reprogramming your mind with positive self-talk!

**What are the negative thoughts
that I need to eliminate?**

_____

_____

_____

"Life is too short to spend in negativity. So I have made a conscious effort to not be where I don't want to be."

-Hugh Dillon

Chapter 8

SURROUND YOURSELF WITH POSTIVE PEOPLE

When the people in your world are positive, you will consistently be in an atmosphere of uplifting stories, exalting affirmations, and inspiring outlooks. Surrounding yourself with negative people will do the exact opposite. Eliminate negative people from your life. They are energy vampires. Negative energy will consume you.

Though they can be hard to find, the positive individual has the ability to focus on the things that give them joy and hope. They feel blessed for the wonderful things that life has given them and do not give much thought to the ways that life has dealt them a bad hand. They tend to see the silver lining in areas where most feel nothing but despair. Learning to be positive will attract positive people to you. Like attracts like. Be a positive person and you will attract positive people.

Rules for Positivity:

1. **Reframe your failures as lessons.**
   We all have imperfections. These imperfections will invariably lead to what most consider failure. As a human being, mistakes will be made and outcomes will not always turn out as we would like. Instead of

thinking about how you failed to get the job done, think about what you are going to do next time to achieve a positive result. Reframe your failure as a lesson. Set up a new game plan and a different approach the next time you are faced with this situation. Analyze the factors that did not work in your favor and devise a way to neutralize them.

2. **Learn to focus on the good things in any situation.**

Almost daily, you will have to deal with unwanted challenges and obstacles. If you think about it, you will find some benefit in dealing with your problem, even though it may be very small. For instance, if you are in a traffic jam you will have a chance to listen to the rest of the audio book you just purchased. If your health food store is out of a particular type of protein powder you regularly use, you will have a chance to try the brand that your buffed friend raves about.

3. **See the humor in negative situations.**

Even in the face of dire circumstances allow yourself to experience humor in the situation. Be open to the fact that an unfortunate occurrence could make for a great story down the line and try to make light of it. I recently told a friend of mine about a dating experience I had with a particular girl as a teenager. It was quite distressing at the time. Looking back at the situation 30 plus years later made for a hilarious story that pretty much had my friend laughing himself to tears!

4. Stay in the Moment.

The majority of negative thoughts and feelings stem from a memory of an unpleasant recent event or exaggerated mental image of what might await in the near future. Learn to focus on the situation you are in right now at this exact moment. You might be getting chewed out by your husband or wife. Don't think about the comment he made ten minutes ago. Don't think about what he/she might say ten minutes from now. Center yourself on this one individual moment in time. What is happening in this exact moment that is so terrible? Most of the time, you will not find it as nearly as horrific as you conceive it to be.

> "Keep your face to the sunshine and you cannot see a shadow."
>
> -Helen Keller

CHAPTER NOTES

Chapter 9

HE'S JUST NOT SMART ENOUGH

When I lived in Savannah, Georgia in the early 1990's, I worked as a salesperson for an extended stay hotel. It was a good job, but I realized that I just wasn't passionate about it. I wanted to impact people's lives and help them in an up close, personal, and positive way. So, after nearly three years in the hotel business, I decided that I would go back to college and become an occupational therapist.

I told all of my friends and most of them were supportive about my decision and offered congratulations and words of encouragement; everyone except a pretty young girl in the operations department named Dawn. Not realizing that I was still in my cubicle, I overhead Dawn really busting my chops. She said, "My mother is a nurse and I know a couple of occupational therapists. I know how tough it is to get through occupational therapy school and how intelligent you need to be to complete the program. Joel just isn't smart enough to make it through OT school." A co-worker named Sean told me that Dawn had shared this thought with others on two other occasions that he knew of.

Now, more committed than ever, I left Savannah to go off to OT school at The University of Louisiana at

Monroe. I would become an occupational therapist. I set my mind. I knew what I wanted. I made it a mission to achieve it no matter what!

Once I got to school, I had to take 36 hours of core courses before the school would accept me into the Occupational Therapy program. This was **IF** I had one of the 30 best GPAs among well over 200 applicants. I was sure I would make it and I had a plan. I was going to make a 4.0 GPA in all of my core courses! I let Dawn's words be part of my motivation. I worked harder and smarter. I stayed focused on the end results that I wanted to achieve and over a three-semester period, I nailed the 4.0!

One usually would have to wait 4-6 weeks or so before they knew if they had made the cut to get into the OT program, but my grades left no doubt; I was a shoe in! After calling several friends and family to tell them the good news, I called Sean at the hotel in Savannah. I told him my good news. He said, "Dawn is right here, let me step up to the front desk and tell her!" On the other end of the phone, I heard Sean report to Dawn that I made a 4.0 on my prerequisites and that "I guess you were wrong that he wasn't smart enough, huh?" Of course, Dawn denied that she ever said it, but Terry let her know that we both remembered what she said about me not achieving my goal. And he rubbed it in her face. I chuckled on the other end of the phone. Dawn was not able to steal my dream!

CHAPTER NOTES

"Never retreat. Never explain. Get it done and let them howl."

-Benjamin Jowett

Chapter 10

MOTIVATION: SOME SIMPLE TIPS

1. Close your eyes, take a deep breath, and visualize yourself reaching your goals.

2. Make a to-do list each morning, scratching items off the list as you complete them.

3. Be sure to get restful sleep. Sleep deprivation is detrimental to being motivated.

4. Begin a proven exercise program.

5. Set a deadline for yourself so you can get a task(s) done before time is up.

6. Play high energy music when performing a task that you really don't want to do to help get you through it.

7. Eat a nutritionally sound diet—you will feel better and your mind will work better.

8. Verbalize your goals to others. This will create internal pressure to get the job done and provide accountability.

9. Don't compare yourself to others. This leads to dis-couragement. Compete against yourself instead.

10. Track your progress toward your goal by journaling. When you can track your progress on paper, you will be motivated to keep going.

11. When you wake up in the morning, immediately think of three things you're grateful for. This will give you emotional momentum for your day.

> "Desire is the key to motivation, but it's determination and commitment to an unre-lenting pursuit of your goal—a commit-ment to excellence—that will enable you to attain the success you seek."
>
> -Mario Andretti

CHAPTER NOTES

_____

_____

_____

_____

Chapter 11

CONCENTRATE TO WIN

Concentration is a skill that develops over time. Being able to block out everything around you and concentrate on the task at hand is a powerful weapon in your mental arsenal. This ability is crucial in attaining virtually any goal.

Pumping iron has been paramount in developing my ability to channel my focus and concentration skills. Through countless hours in the gym, intense concentration attainment has had a powerful positive carryover effect. Having the skills to concentrate and focus has allowed me to conquer a plethora of goals in other aspects of my life.

Abilities developed through my love for bodybuilding and weight lifting has literally changed the course of my existence. Aspects of my positive experiences in human development go all the way back to what I learned in the gym during my teenage years. This is why each time I go to hit the iron, I am excited knowing that I will enhance my ability to concentrate, to achieve, to conquer!

"Concentration comes out of a combination of confidence and hunger."

-Arnold Palmer

What areas of my life will be enhanced by improved concentration skills?

_____

_____

_____

_____

_____

_____

_____

_____

_____

_____

_____

_____

Chapter 12

BUILDING SELF-ESTEEM FOR A HEALTHIER MIND AND BODY

Self-esteem is the hallmark of mental health. High self-esteem sets you up for a well-rounded and happy life as well as giving you the foundation to acquire your goals and dreams. If you have low self-esteem, chances of success in any endeavor will be limited. A few simple tips for overcoming low self-esteem can truly make a difference:

HELP OTHERS

When we consistently focus on our fellow man, magic happens. Doing selfless things for others with the expectation of not receiving anything back is a reward within itself. It builds confidence and makes you feel good about who you are. Try to do something special and selflessly help someone once a week and see what happens!

KEEP THE RIGHT COMPANY

Make time to be with people that care about you and appreciate who you are. Eliminate relationships with negative people. They are an energy drain and will end up making you feel as miserable as they are. They will tear you down. Spend time with individuals who lift you up and have positive energy!

SET DAILY GOALS FOR YOURSELF

Write a set of goals and/or tasks to achieve each morning upon awakening. As you go through your day scratch items off the list as you complete them. You will have a significant feeling of satisfaction when you see everything on your list scratched off by the end of the day!

LEARN TO RELAX

Stress can be very destructive to self-esteem. Being able to combat stress is vital to self-esteem maintenance. Each day find something to do that is relaxing. This could be taking a soothing bath in a dark room with candles lit all around you, listening to classical music while kicking back in your recliner, etc. Do whatever it takes to relax at some point each day!

EAT WELL, EXERCISE WELL

Eating nutritious food along with consistent exercise boosts endorphins, which are the body's natural opiates. You will feel good about yourself when you know you are doing what is right for your body!

VISUALIZE VICTORY

If your mind can conceive it, you can achieve it. Write down your goals. Each day, write down 3 action steps that you can take which will move you closer to achieving your goals. Each day take time to set aside 3 minutes for *VISUALIZATION*. Close your eyes, take 3 deep breaths and see yourself performing at your very best —looking your very best—FEELING your very best! Feel the excitement rush through your body during the visualization. Entrenching this emotion in your physical body during the visualization will convince your subconscious that the visualization is real. See a clear picture of what and who you want to be. Take the needed action steps to make it happen and SEE IT in your mind's eye until it becomes real!

CHAPTER NOTES

_____

_____

_____

_____

_____

_____

_____

Chapter 13

HOW TO GIVE YOUR GOALS POWER

Make long-term and short-term goals for everything that you really want to accomplish. Write your goals down. Look at them frequently and develop a plan to attain them. Having goals gives you the roadmap to achieving success. So many guys/gals go to the gym with the goal only to work hard or "get a pump." However, these goals are not specific enough to create real progress. Your goal must be very specific with a timetable/deadline to reach your goal.

Make your long-term goal first, then make short-term goals that will lead the way to attaining your long-term goal. Will you reach a new destination without a map? Make goals to reach your ultimate potential!

What is my 10-year goal?

_____

_____

_____

_____

**What are the yearly and daily goals
that will get me there?**

_____

_____

_____

_____

_____

_____

_____

_____

_____

_____

"Setting goals is the first step in turning the
invisible into the visible."

-Tony Robbins

Chapter 14

PAIN IS TEMPORARY...
QUITTING IS FOREVER

Quitting does not take any talent or a particular set of skills. Anyone can do it. Repeated failures or discouraging words from others can make you feel like quitting. But don't give in—persist.

Some people like nothing better than destroying another person's belief in themselves. They derive a high from cutting you down. You have two choices: You can let their intended discouragement make you quit, or you could keep going, believe in yourself, and eventually reach your goals.

Many of us have heard that we don't have what it takes; that we will never amount to much. My question to you is when you are 80 years old, are you going to have the regret of quitting on something that could have made your life better if you had persisted? I personally want to die with no regrets. Don't give up on your dreams and goals, and you won't die with many regrets either!

So many of us quit when we are unknowingly on the brink of a huge victory. Don't be the person that does this. Keep pushing toward your goal even if it seems like it is more than arms-length away. Also, be open to changing your approach if what you are doing is not working. Write down your goals. Look at them daily. Visualize attaining them. Feel it. Do it!

What are the "tough to achieve" goals that you will not quit on until you achieve them?

_____

_____

_____

_____

_____

_____

_____

"Don't quit. Never give up on trying to build the world you can see, even if others can't see it. Listen to your drum and your drum only. It's the only one that makes the sweetest sound."

-Simon Sinek

Chapter 15

THE STORY OF CAROL

"You are not college material."

One of my all-time favorite personal training clients has a fantastic story illustrating how the underdog can achieve victory over the naysayer; about how we must press on despite those who try to steal our dreams. Her name is Carol Edwards.

Carol always knew she would go to college and have a career as a professional in the education field. This was ingrained in her by her parents and it was something that she wanted very much for herself as well. In her mind, not going to college was **never** an option. She would earn her degree and be successful in her chosen profession; **no** doubt about it!

Carol was in her junior year of high school in 1966. She wanted information on how to apply for college in her home state of Michigan, so she set up an appointment with the counselor at her high school, Mr. Burns. As she walked in to Mr. Burn's office, she had no idea of the "cold cup of coffee" she was about to get from him.

After greeting each other, they sat down and Carol stated that all she was really looking to do was get help from Mr. Burns in the college application process. Mr. Burns asked, "Have you taken the SAT?" Carol replied that she had. Mr. Burns looked through his files and found Carol's SAT results. Mr. Burns asked, "Can you type?" Carol replied that she could and that it was part of her college prep curriculum. Mr. Burns told Carol, "It is good that you can type. Secretarial school may be an option for you, but I don't see you making it in college. You will probably get married in a couple of years anyway, so you will have a husband to take care of you." Carol simply replied, "Well, sir, that is not my plan." She stood up and quietly walked out of Mr. Burn's office, but the inside of her burned with both rage and determination.

Four years after Carol graduated high school, she earned her bachelor's degree from a nearby state college. Mr. Burn's assessment that Carol was not college material ended up being dead wrong. Carol was going to make sure that Mr. Burns knew this! She wanted him to know that he was not successful in negatively determining her destiny.

Carol called her old high school and asked if Mr. Burns still worked there. Sure enough, he did. Same place, same position as a high school counselor. Carol told the secretary that she was a former student that Mr. Burns had advised and she just wanted a few minutes of his time to discuss something. The secretary set up an appointment for the two to meet.

On the day of the appointment, Carol was eager and determined to "drop the bomb" on Mr. Burns. As Carol walked in to Mr. Burn's office, she introduced herself by saying, "You probably don't remember me, but I was a student you once advised. My name is Carol Edwards. You told me I wasn't college material. You told me to forget college, use my typing skills to become a secretary, and to find a husband to take care of me. I wonder how many other young women you misled like this?" (Remember, this was the 1960's, where a lot of guys thought a woman's place was in the kitchen—barefoot and pregnant). "Well, I would like to present you with my bachelor's degree that comes from someone who you told was not college material.

Mr. Burns just stood there and didn't know what to say. He looked dumbfounded and appeared to be totally at a loss for words. Carol ended the silence with a nice, polite, "Have a nice day" and walked out of Mr. Burn's office. This time, however, Carol did not walk away with rage and determination; she walked away with satisfaction and victory.

An inaccurate assessment by a male chauvinist did not adversely affect her life in the way it probably did for countless other young women at Carol's high school. It instead created more fuel for success. Again, this illustrates how much we need to believe in ourselves when others do not; even if they are "experts" or "authorities." Carol would not allow herself to be discouraged by someone's inaccurate assessment of her potential; and hundreds of young men and women that she has taught the last 30 plus years are much better because of it!

Chapter 16

ACTING "AS IF": YOUR IDEAL SELF

What is the "As If" principle? It is simply a principle that allows us to create our outer circumstances by acting "As If" they were already a reality. For example, we can become happy by acting as if we ARE happy.

To utilize this principle, start off by imagining the aspects of your ideal self. This could entail being an incredibly successful entrepreneur, being in the physical shape of your life, or being a great parent.

Next, think of an obstacle you're facing in one of these areas where you are procrastinating in doing what needs to be done. You become discouraged about your entrepreneurship, you have eaten poorly the last few days, you have added a few pounds on the scale and you just don't feel like going to the gym now. Your kids are driving you crazy, and you just feel like yelling at them instead of becoming parent of the year. Now, as you experience these negative feelings, take a second and imagine your IDEAL SELF and contemplate how that version of you would step up and handle these feelings and problems.

Your ideal self would take a deep breath and imagine the payoff of taking the actions needed to become a successful entrepreneur and move forward on them at this moment. Your actions would then lead you to head to the gym with determination to have an incredible workout! You would resist the temptation to rip into your kids and apply methods you just learned in a particular parenting article to perfection.

That is basically all there is to it. The next time you are feeling like less than the ultimate version of yourself when faced with these feelings and situations, think about how your IDEAL SELF would handle them and act as if you ALREADY WERE this big-time version of you! It takes a little practice, but it is worth the effort.

**In what ways will you become
YOUR IDEAL SELF?**

_____

_____

_____

_____

> "In our society, the ideal self is bold, gregarious, and comfortable in the spotlight. We like to think that we value individuality, but mostly we admire the type of individual who's comfortable putting himself out there."
>
> -Susan Cain

Chapter 17

GIVE YOUR BEST EFFORT

Strong Effort = Success

Why would you ever give less than your best effort on anything? Your subconscious cannot be lied to because it knows when you are giving less than your best. This leads to you not feeling as well about life as you could. Your self-esteem and self-image suffer when you continually do things halfway.

When you consistently give strong effort in all that you do, your subconscious feels much better about who you are. The results are that you help yourself succeed much more as well as have a positive effect on those around you. Give your best at all times, whether it be your workouts, your education, or your job. You know what needs to be done, now go do it well!

**In what ways am I hurting myself
by not giving my best effort?**

_____

_____

_____

_____

"With hard work and effort, you can achieve anything."

-Antoine Griezmann

Chapter 18

EMBRACE THE HATE

It is a jealous world. For every two people who rejoice in your victories, there will be an individual who burns with jealousy over your achievements. My father once told me with his thick Arkansas drawl, "Son, people will forgive you for most anything except for success." I often questioned what I thought was my father's cynicism, only to learn later he was pretty much on the money with his analysis.

There will be those who despise you because of your attainment of high achievement. There are those who will be thrilled for your success as well. Just know that success is a double-edged sword. If you are successful, THERE WILL BE HATERS! Understand that if you sometimes get doused with "haterade" it is because you have probably succeeded at a high level. You are being hated on for doing something RIGHT instead of doing something wrong, in all likelihood. Do not acquiesce to make haters feel better. Kick butt and take names!

Also, accept that there will be plenty of friends who will be happy for you as you journey to the top! Those that will not be happy for you are probably having issues with self-image and self-esteem, so don't necessarily take them personally. Just keep on rising above it all and succeeding, whether it be in the boardroom, in your relationships, or in the gym!

List 3 pre-determined positive statements that you will use when someone expresses jealousy or hate towards you.

_____

_____

_____

_____

_____

_____

_____

_____

> "People who hate you because of mere jealousy over your success hurt themselves in disguise. This is because you carry an image of who they wish they had become."
> -Israelmore Ayivor

Chapter 19

THERE IS NO ONE LIKE YOU!

Be your unique self, don't feel like you have to be any-one else. Borrowing from a Billy Joel song, "Don't go changing to try to please me…" If people don't dig you for who you are, the heck with them. This can especially be true if you are an achiever or someone who dreams and strives for lofty goals. Haters will try to discourage you and/or hate you because they do not have the intestinal fortitude to do the same. Don't lower yourself to their level of mediocrity by trying to make them feel better via stifling your energy. Reach for the sky, follow your dream, and be yourself, no matter what anyone else thinks!

In what ways am I positively unique?

_____

_____

_____

_____

_____

"I find that the very things I get criticized for, which is usually being different and just doing my own thing and just being original, is the very thing that's making me success-ful."

-Shania Twain

Chapter 20

DON'T BE A JIMMY OR A DICK

Some people are afraid of real challenges or of a situation where they are not guaranteed to win. We need to go for the things we really desire in life despite the possibility of failure. No guts, no glory.

The following story took place in the early 1990's in Savannah, Georgia and is about about myself and two guys I will call Jimmy and Dick. Jimmy was really a nice guy. Dick was—well, let's just say that I gave him the proper alias for this story.

One evening I saw a flyer advertising two body-building contests that would be held on the same night: the Mr. Savannah and Mr. Adonis competitions. The Savannah was a local show open only to residents of Chatham County (the 5th largest county in Georgia). There were seven gyms at the time in Savannah. Being a beach town, there were some formidable bodies walking the sands of nearby Tybee Island. The Adonis was for anyone from anywhere. That particular year, Mr. Adonis drew competitors from as far away as Clemson, SC and Jacksonville, FL. However, I'd previously performed very well in higher level shows than these. My interest was minimal, until my encounter with Dick.

Dick was a brash, rude, arrogant kid who was about 22 years old at the time. I would often get nasty glances from the guy, which I would later learn was born of his insecurities. He was working the front desk one night at the gym as I walked through the front door. I noticed that he was eating fish and a baked potato with broccoli. Dick had a good physique; he was very lean and symmetrical. I assumed that he was preparing for one of the bodybuilding competitions. I politely asked him "Hey man, it looks like you are getting ready for something. What show are you getting ready for?" Without moving his head from over his plate or even giving me the courtesy of eye contact, Dick deadpanned with his thick southern drawl "The Savannah." I remember thinking, "Holy cow! What a tool!"

Jimmy was an energetic, seemingly confident and very friendly fellow. With his small joints that flared into large muscle bellies highlighted by his ebony skin, Jimmy was a truly natural genetic freak. Jimmy was bombing his chest and back while I was working out with my friend Stuart. I told Stuart, "Jimmy over there looks like a real bodybuilder. He has some serious muscle!" Stuart replied, "I think he is getting ready for the Mr. Savannah; Joel, you should enter this contest. I have seen it the last three years and none of the winners were in the shape you are in RIGHT NOW! You would smoke any of the guys that I have seen win this contest!" I could tell Stuart was shooting me straight. As I watched Jimmy train out of the corner of my eye, I noticed that my body fat level was significantly lower than his. I believed that my muscle shape and symmetry were at least as good as Jimmy's. I also thought that a chance to put a rear-end kicking on Dick was appealing too! Right then and there, I told Stuart, "I'm going to do it!"

After I saw that Jimmy was finished with his work-out, I walked up to him and told him how great he looked. He was very polite and appreciative. I asked, "Jimmy, are you going to compete in the Savannah and the Adonis?" Jimmy replied, "Oh yeah! The Savannah for sure! I'm working hard for it!" I said, "Awesome— so am I!" The smile on Jimmy's face quickly dissipated. Jimmy managed to get out an unconvincing "Oh, cool" with a face that could not feign his concern. I got the feeling that someone had told Jimmy what Stuart had told me—that he was a shoe-in to win. Now that feeling of certain victory had turned into serious doubt in light of the new obstacle that stood before him. The next morning, I turned in my paperwork and entry fee for the contest.

The very next night, I walked into the gym for my first workout as an official competitor for the contest and guess who was working the front desk? The ever-so-pleasant Dick! It was time for me to drop the bomb on him. His gazes of hatred and disrespect towards me were about to be paid back in spades! "What's up, brother?" I said with no attempt to hide my sarcasm. He peeked up at me from his plate of chicken and sweet potato with no response.

I put both hands on the desk and slowly leaned in towards Dick's smug face. "I'm entering the Savannah and the Adonis with you. It's going to be great to be up there onstage representing this gym with you and Jimmy!" Dick's face dropped like he had just received news that Ms. Georgia had broken up with him. It was the look of a man whose hopes had just died. And they did. I found out a couple of days later that Dick had decided not to enter for some reason that he wasn't talking about, but I knew what it was. I am sure that he knew that I knew what it was. Bang! I really wanted to defeat Dick on the stage. However, Dick beat himself by shrinking in the face of possible defeat.

Jimmy was going to be my main competition in the The Savannah. I was pretty sure that a couple of guys might show up from nowhere and push me in the Adonis, but I would not know who they were until the day of the show. However, I felt that if Jimmy could really dial in on his condition a bit in the last three weeks, I would have my hands full with him. I practiced my posing in those last three weeks like a man possessed. Every morsel of food I put in my mouth was weighed and measured. I perfectly nailed my target heart rate each time I did cardio, and I trained on the weights till I dropped as I envisioned being on stage with an in-shape Jimmy. The idea of competing against him really pushed me to become better. Unfortunately, Jimmy's idea of competing against me had the opposite effect. I ran into him in the gym exactly two weeks prior to the contest. I asked him "Jimmy, how is the pre-contest prep going?" "It's over." replied Jimmy. "I just don't have enough time between now and the show to get in the condition I need to be in."

I went on to win both the Mr. Savannah and Mr. Adonis in convincing fashion. Soon after, a common friend relayed to me the more precise reason for Jimmy's withdrawal. He said, "There was no way I was going to be able to beat that ripped dude from New Orleans." Jimmy allowed himself to be defeated the day I told him I would be competing against him. I still think that I would have beaten him if we had both showed up at our best.

But what if I caught a stomach bug a few days before the contest that would keep me from being at my peak on stage? (This exact thing happened to me a year later, costing me the overall title at the NPC Dixie Championships.) Jimmy could have beaten me if I had showed up slightly off the mark. However, he chose not to show up, thus not positioning himself to win in case I had a bad day. Bodybuilding, like in all other sports, can take unexpected turns on the day of the event. That is why you have to **SHOW UP AND PLAY THE GAME**! You never know with certainty what can happen. If you are passionate about something, don't give up. Virtually every weekend during football season, an underdog somewhere pulls the big upset over a more talented opponent. You must show up and fight no matter how much the odds are stacked against you.

To his credit, Jimmy recovered and won the Mr. Savannah two years later and placed 3rd in the Mr. Adonis. (In a 2016 conversation with Savannah bodybuilding legend Mark Lynn, I was told that no one has won both shows on the same night since I accomplished the feat 25 years before in 1991). Jimmy later on won a big drug-tested national title in California which I found out about while watching a bodybuilding program on ESPN. As for Dick, I'm not sure what ever happened to him. It is my hope that he didn't continue to duck and cover when life presented him its challenges.

THE BOTTOM LINE IS THIS:

The things that you will regret at the end of your life are not areas where you attempted and failed, but the things that you failed to attempt. Don't cower and run when you face a situation that will not be an automatic win. Where is the glory in an easy victory? Go after what you want in life without being paralyzed by the obstacles. Without losses in life, you cannot appreciate the wins! If you give full effort with a strong game plan that is well thought out, you will be able to accept the result, whatever it is. Don't be the person that says "I wish I woulda, I wish I coulda, I think I shoulda." Remember that the person that never loses is the person that never plays the game.

> "Under any circumstance, simply do your best, and you will avoid self judgement, self - abuse, and regret."
>
> -Don Miguel Ruiz

Chapter 21

THE STORY OF "HOSSMAN" - Never Say Die!

Mark "Hossman" Allen is one the most inspirational people that I have ever known. I met Mark one day at Shultze Cafeteria on the campus of The University of Louisiana—Monroe in 1984. What I first noticed about Mark was his outgoing personality and his unique "southern gentleman" aura. What I did not pick up on right away was the fire that burned inside of him—his tenacity, his resilience, his inability to ever give up on anything important to him. I would get to know that about Mark as the years passed and his greatness became more and more evident.

Mark was about 5' 11" inches tall and weighed about 145 pounds. His frame was very slight. It was not a physique that appeared very athletic, much less a physique that would ever make it in the world of competitive bodybuilding. It did not take Mark long to decide that he wanted to become a bodybuilding champion.

Mark and I worked out together for less than a year before he entered his first bodybuilding contest. Mark competed in the 1985 Southern Mississippi body-building championship and won a well-deserved 2nd place. He was happy, but still wanted more. Mark would always tell me, "Big Joel, I am going to win the next time." Mark never doubted that he would become a champion. However, that bodybuilding win that Mark longed for would be very elusive.

For the next nine years, Mark would enter a contest every year; he would finish 2nd or 3rd place every time. It appeared that he would never achieve his dream. Most individuals I know would have thrown in the towel after half of the tough losses that Mark had faced. I remember him calling me before the 1996 Mississippi bodybuilding championships. "Big Joel, I've got this one; this is my time." To borrow a phrase from Tony Robbins, Mark always believed, "The past does not equal the future." Ten years of 2nd and 3rd place finishes did not mean to him that he was going to come up short this time. He saw himself as a champion, and he became one.

On a hot night in Jackson, MS, Mark "Hossman" Allen won the 1996 NPC Mississippi Bodybuilding Championship!

"Failure will never overtake me if my determination to succeed is strong enough."
-Og Mandino

CHAPTER NOTES

_____

_____

_____

_____

_____

_____

_____

_____

_____

_____

_____

_____

_____

Chapter 22

HOW JOHN CURED STUTTERING BY PUMPING IRON

When I was in college in the 1980s, there was a young fellow at my gym that we will call "John." John was a nice guy, but obviously did not have a lot of confidence. He also had a significant speech impediment and could hardly utter a sentence without stuttering. Somehow, this was a problem that was never addressed with John in the public school system with a speech pathologist. He was about 19 years old when I met him and would stutter without fail each time I talked with him. As a newbie to pumping iron, he would be what you would call a "skinny fat guy." John had very small arms and legs and a significant amount of fat around his midsection.

After a few months of lifting on his own, Jim somehow connected with a group of very knowledgeable powerlifters. He soon started training with them. He packed on a lot of muscle in a very brief period of time (I'm pretty sure there was much more than simply pumping iron involved in his rapid progress). Nonetheless, his feats of strength in the gym as well as his physique became quite impressive.

As the son of a speech pathologist, I noticed another incredible improvement in John: HE BARELY STUTTERED ANYMORE! The confidence he gained from working out allowed him to now look you in the eye when he talked to you. John now brimmed with confidence. He now had strength, a very impressive physique, and probably the first girlfriend that he ever had.

Everything had changed. John saw himself in a different way and his life underwent a metamorphosis. I believe that the confidence he gained through his effort in the gym changed all aspects of his life; including having so much confidence that it became his cure for stuttering!

"To feel strong, to walk amongst humans with a tremendous feeling of confidence and superiority is not at all wrong. The sense of superiority in bodily strength is born out of the long history of mankind paying homage in folklore, song, and poetry to strong men."
-Fred Hatfield

Chapter 23

THE MOTIVATED AND FIT WEIGHT TRAINING SYSTEM

The Motivated and Fit Weight Training System is based around the concept of ABBREVIATED TRAINING. Abbreviated training is a minimalist approach to weight training. This usually consists of pumping iron no more than 2 or 3 days a week on just a handful of exercises. Overall training volume is much less than what is usually found in today's weight training programs. It is a very simple, structured style of lifting based on consistency and a focus on poundage progression utilizing basic multi-joint movements.

Abbreviated training is the best way to make true progress for the vast majority of individuals. It is a methodology that helps keep one from overtraining, which has been a plague in the fitness world for decades. Overtraining is the biggest reason there is so much failure for most to make progress in the gym. Rapid turnover of gym memberships would not be the norm if sensible training routines (abbreviated) were used by the resistance training universe.

Many make the mistake of trying to emulate the routines of Mr. or Ms. Olympia or maybe the most physically impressive guy/woman in the gym. Chances are, their routines will not work for you. This is because they are more than likely genetic superiors and/or performance enhancement drug assisted. Don't waste hours, days, months, and years attempting to train in a way for you that is non-productive.

Most of you will benefit much more by making use of training methods which were espoused in the pre-steroid era (prior to 1960). The training advice at that time was much more applicable to the general population than what is available today. Resolve NOW to not waste time and spend it on realistic training principles that have been proven and time tested. A lifestyle for training that will work for the masses is what I will be presenting to you.

"For the production of best-possible results, every possible effort must be made in the direction of progress—and if this is done properly, then at least some sign of progress will be seen in almost every workout."

-Arthur Jones

Chapter 24

THE MOTIVATED AND FIT BEGINNER WORKOUT

(Progression Phase One)

Each phase builds upon the other. Beginners or those that have not been involved with resistance training in a while should begin with *Progression Phase One*. No one seems to be able to definitively agree on who invented the system that will be described in *Progression Phase One*. Much evidence suggests that the man first responsible for this may have been Bob Hoffman back in the 1940's with the book, *Simplified System of Barbell Training*. This phase will create what I call the progress habit. The body and mind will get so accustomed to making measurable increases in workload each session that you will always expect progress and look forward to every workout! You will perform your workouts on 3 non-consecutive days per week. This could be Monday, Wednesday, Friday OR Tuesday, Thursday, Saturday OR whatever days work best for your schedule.

Here are the rules for *Progression Phase One*:

I.   Perform no more than 8 exercises. We want to start out nice and easy. Your first routine will be made up of the following exercises:

1. Barbell Bench Press
2. Barbell Overhead Press
3. Bent Over Barbell Row
4. Barbell Curl
5. Barbell Squat
6. Deadlift
7. Calf Raise
8. Crunch Sit Up

II. Initially, you will perform only one set of each of the above exercises.

III. In your first workout, perform 5 repetitions on exercises 1-6, and 10 repetitions on exercises 7 and 8. Start off with a weight that you could perform 8 or 9 repetitions with on exercises 1-6; start off with a weight you could perform 16 or 18 repetitions with on exercises 7 and 8. Again, we want to start off nice and easy and establish forward momentum.

IV. Add 1 repetition each workout on exercises 1-6 and 2 repetitions each workout on exercises 7 and 8.

V. Continue to add repetitions each workout until you *double* the amount of repetitions on each exercise that you started with. This means you would now be doing 10 repetitions on exercises 1-6 and 20 repetitions on exercises 7 and 8.

VI. At this point, add 5-10 lbs. on the Barbell Bench Press, the Barbell Overhead Press, the Bent Over Barbell Row, the Barbell Squat, and the Deadlift. These are the "big exercises" where larger weight increases are possible. You can also add 5-10 lbs. on the Calf Raise. Add 2.5 to 5 lbs. on the Barbell Curl and Crunch Sit Up.

*NOTE: How to make the 2.5 pound increase will be explained later in this chapter.

Weight can be added on the Crunch Sit Up by holding a barbell plate or a dumbbell/kettlebell at the chest. Alternatively, if you find holding a weight at the chest uncomfortable or inconvenient, you can just continue to add 2 repetitions each workout until you reach 30 repetitions. Once you reach 30 repetitions, don't add any more repetitions in the upcoming workouts. More volume to the ab workouts will be added later.

VII. With the weights on each exercise now increased, drop your repetitions back down to 5 reps on exercises 1-6 and 10 reps on exercises 7 and 8. (See above about possible exception on exercise 8).

VIII. Repeat this cycle 4 more times for a total of 5 cycles. Add reps until they are doubled, and again add weight. You will be amazed at the strength increase you will have at this point!

The squat illustrates the effectiveness of *Progression Phase One:* A trainee who was squatting 1 x 5 with 120 lbs. in his first workout will be squatting 1 x 5 with 150 lbs. in just over two months based on a 10-pound increment at the end of three cycles. Five cycles would produce a squat of 1 x 5 with 170 pounds. NOW, THAT IS SERIOUS PROGRESS!

After you have performed 5 cycles utilizing one set per exercise, you will increase your training volume by performing two sets of each exercise. This will be the second stage of *Progression Phase One*. Your workout will now be:

1. Barbell Bench Press: 2 sets of 5 reps (2x5)
2. Barbell Overhead Press: 2 sets of 5 reps(2x5)
3. Bent Over Barbell Row: 2 sets of 5 reps (2x5)
4. Barbell Curl: 2 sets of 5 reps (2x5)
5. Barbell Squat: 2 sets of 5 reps (2x5)
6. Deadlift: 2 sets of 5 reps (2x5)
7. Calf Raise: 2 sets of 10 reps (2x10)
8. Crunch Sit Up: 2 sets of 10-30 reps (2x10-30)

The second stage of Progression Phase One works just like the one set portion of the program. Work your way up to doubling the reps on each exercise, add weight, drop the reps back down, then work your way back up. At this point in the program you will benefit from doing two warm up sets of five reps with approximately 45% and 50% of the weight you will be using for each exercise. Injury prevention through warm up is very important. Rest 3 to 4 minutes between sets. Be sure to give the body time to recuperate from the previous set. You will be using some considerably heavy weight at this point in the program. The muscles must be recuperated to fire with maximal force in each set that is performed. Don't turn your workout into a cardio or endurance event. Train slow, train steady, build muscle!

After five cycles of two sets, it will be time to move up to a three set per exercise protocol. This part of the program really raises the exercise volume and the work performed by the muscular system.

This third and final stage of *Progressive Phase One* works just like the previous two stages. The only difference is that you will now be doing three sets per exercise. After five cycles of the three-set protocol, you will have literally transformed into a NEW PERSON from where you started! The final stage of this phase is as follows:

1. Barbell Bench Press: 3 sets of 5 reps (3x5)
2. Barbell Overhead Press: 3 sets of 5 reps (3x5)
3. Bent Over Barbell Row: 3 sets of 5 reps (3x5)
4. Barbell Curl: 3 sets of 5 reps (3x5)
5. Barbell Squat: 3 sets of 5 reps (3x5)
6. Deadlift: 3 sets of 5 reps (3x5)
7. Calf Raise: 3 sets of 10 reps (3x10)
8. Crunch Sit up: 3 sets of 10-30 reps (3x10-30)

FRACTIONAL WEIGHT PLATES

Fractional weight plates are a tool needed to make 2.5 pound progressions. The average gym and common Olympic barbell weight set do not have plates small enough to make a 2.5 pound weight increment. The smallest plates they have are 2.5 pound plates which means that the smallest weight jumps you can make are usually 5 pounds. Fractional weight plates allow you to basically make any weight increment you desire. A set of fractional weights will have pairs of .25 pounds, .50 pounds, .75 pounds, and 1 pound plates. They can be purchased as set on Amazon or other sellers for about $45 U.S. dollars a set. You will need all of them training *The Motivated and Fit* way moving forward. You will need the 1 pound and .25 pound plates to make the 2.5 pound progressions needed on some exercises in *Progression Phase One*. The other plates will be needed in the intermediate and advanced progression phases to make variable small weight increases from workout to workout.

"Dream more than others think practical. Expect more than others think possible."
-Frank Zane

Chapter 25

THE MOTIVATED AND FIT INTERMEDIATE WORKOUT

(Intermediate Progression Phase)

The Intermediate Progression Phase is where every workout is a challenge. Being considerably stronger after completing *Progression Phase One*, your strength increases will slow down a bit. You will have to be happy with small bits of strength training progress at a time. From workout to workout, it will be unusual to increase the weight of any of our exercises more than 5 lbs. at a time. Now is the time to put all of your .25, .50, and .75 pound fractional weight plates in your gym bag! VERY SMALL WEIGHT INCREASES at this stage are ideal for a number of reasons.

Reasons include:

1. Adding too much weight to the bar too quickly at the intermediate level can cause you to "stall out" your progress. You can make too big of a weight jump which can cause your *progress habit* to experience failure by not successfully handling the new weight.

2. Adding too much weight to the bar too quickly before the body is prepared to handle it can

quickly lead to injury! Injury can sideline you for months!

3. Small weight increases can be virtually *imperceptible* to the intermediate trainee!

Consider the following example: A very strong intermediate female can deadlift 200 lbs. for 1 x 5. Instead of trying to increase the weight too quickly, she takes what I call the slow cooking approach. She sneaks up on the poundage progression by adding a pound a week on the deadlift using fractional weight plates. If her last deadlift session felt really light, she might add as much as 2.5 lbs. at her next workout. If this trainee adds an average of one pound a week over the course of a year, she is now deadlifting 252 lbs. for 1 x 5. That is a gain of 52 lbs. for 5 reps in a year. HUGE PROGRESS! If eating correctly was implemented along with this type of progress in the gym, how different will her body look? Now being able to deadlift 52 pounds more for 1 x 5, she will look much more tight, toned, and sexy!

The Intermediate Progression Phase focuses on what is called the 3 x 5 system; 3 sets of 5 reps are performed on the majority of exercises in this phase (the exception in this phase being calves and abdominals where more reps will be utilized). The 5-rep set system became popular back in the 1950's where English bodybuilder Reg Park utilized it to become Mr. Universe in 1951, 1958, and 1965. In the 1970's, strength coach Bill Starr put his 5 x 5 system on display and received much notoriety for his program in the book *The Strongest Shall Survive*.

In the early 90s, as I began to study abbreviated training, I started to use much more sensible routines based on poundage progression with the focus being 3x5 sets with heavy weights. Being a natural body-builder, I figured out that I could not tolerate the volume of work that was being propagated by the popular muscle magazines of that time. Thus, training in a manner that the superstars of the pre-steroid era utilized was what I emulated. 3x5 sets seemed to have been what many of the best of this era used, so I figured I'd give it a try.

I improved my body with this system like I had never done with any other system. As a personal trainer, I have used it with both men and women with great success. It will work for virtually anyone. The routine for the *Intermediate Progression Phase is the following:*

MONDAY:
1. Barbell Bench Press: 3 sets of 5 reps (3x5)
2. Bent Over Barbell Row or Lat Pull Down: 3 sets of 5 reps (3x5)
3. Squat: 3 sets of 5 reps (3x5)
4. Romanian Deadlift: 3 sets of 5 reps (3x5)
5. Barbell Shrug: 3 sets of 5 reps (3x5)
6. Hanging Leg Raise: 3 sets of 15 reps (3x15)

THURSDAY:
1. Barbell Overhead Press: 3 sets of 5 reps (3x5)
2. Trap Bar Deadlift: 3 sets of 5 (3x5)
3. Close Grip Bench Press: 3 sets of 5 reps (3x5)

4. Barbell Curl: 3 sets of 5 reps (3x5)
5. Calf Raise: 3 sets of 15 reps (3x15)
6. Weighted Crunch: 3 sets of 15 reps (3x15)

Monday and Thursday are listed as training days, but one can train any two days per week as long as there is two or three days of rest in between workouts. The *Intermediate Progression Phase* utilizes what is called a *divided workout*. Unlike in *Progression Phase One*, different exercises are performed in the two workouts. More exercises are added to the routine, but they are split up over two workouts.

With the strength increases that were made in Progression Phase One, warm up sets become more critical. Warm up sets can be tricky; they can't be so heavy that they interfere with the weight used on your heavy 3 x 5 sets, but should be just heavy enough to where sufficient resistance is applied to have the proper warm up effect.

A percentage system to prepare for the 3 x 5 sets seems to work best. The following is a breakdown on what a trainee using 225 lbs. for 3x5 on the bench press would look like:

1. Warm up set 1: bar x 5 reps, 45 lbs.
2. Warm up set 2: 45% x 5 reps, 100 lbs.
3. Warm up set 3: 50% x 3 reps, 112.5 lbs.
4. Warm up set 4: 60% x 2 reps, 135 lbs.

*Working sets: 3 x 5, 225 lbs.

Warm up sets allow you to practice the movement of the exercise before the weight becomes heavy. The lighter weights allow preparation of the movement pattern so when the weight gets heavy, you simply focus on pushing hard instead of thinking about how to push.

Four warm up sets may seem like a lot, but you can move through these sets fairly quickly. You only need to take 1-2 minutes between each warm up set. The exceptions to this warm up protocol are for the hanging leg raise, weighted crunch, and the calf raise. The hanging leg raise is performed with body weight only, so no warm up is applicable. The weighted crunch and calf raise require only one warm up set at about 60% of your 3 x 15 weight.

On your 3 x 5 sets, you will be working hard. You want to use a weight that is challenging, but not impossible. Ideally, after all three sets are performed, you should feel like you could have used 1 pound to 5 pounds more. This is where poundage progression becomes an art. Take notes on the weights used and how much more weight you think you could have done. This can be done on a fitness app, written down in a composition notebook, etc.

In my own training, I take notes on the weight used in each exercise as well as how difficult or easy the weight was in performing my 3 x 5 sets. If I felt I could have used five more pounds with an absolute maximum effort, I might add just 2.5 pounds to the bar at my next workout. If there are any secrets to progression, this is one of them! Work hard but always leave just a bit left in the tank. The next time add just a little more weight.

Allow your body to make an adaptive response and get stronger. Use the fractional weight plates to slowly, steadily progress the weight on you 3 x 5 sets. Again, adding too much weight will simply stall your progress. Poundage greed will also cause you to use a weight that your muscles, tendons, and ligaments are simply not ready for which will lead to injury.

Don't let the term "intermediate" fool you! The *Intermediate Progression Phase* is what I utilize probably 60% of the time. I am 54 years old and have been training with weights for over 40 years. Most would consider me "advanced;" however, this training methodology and workout volume will suit a lifter of considerable experience quite well. This phase can be used for months at a time. Just take care to maintain your *progression habit* by making the small poundage increases that have been discussed. When progress finally stalls, it will be time to move to another program for a while. Until then, remember something that I used to read that hung on my grandmother's kitchen wall: "Yard by yard, life is hard; inch by inch, life's a cinch!"

The Three-Day Divided Schedule Option

The *Motivated and Fit Intermediate Program* is based upon two resistance training workouts per week. However, some people enjoy the weight room so much that they had rather train three days per week. Others had rather utilize three days a week due to feeling overtrained by performing six tough exercises in the two workout per week format. The three-day divided schedule option works better for a lot of trainees. The same twelve exercises that are in the two day per week plan are simply redistributed over the week so only four exercises are performed each session. It looks like the following:

Monday:

1. Bench Press: 3 sets of 5 reps (3x5)
2. Bent Over Barbell Row or Lat Pulldown: 3 sets of 5 reps (3x5)
3. Calf Raise: 3 sets of 15 reps (3x15)
4. Hanging Leg Raise: 3 sets of 15 reps (3x15)

Wednesday:

1. Barbell Overhead Press: 3 sets of 5 reps (3x5)
2. Trap Bar Deadlift: 3 sets of 5 reps (3x5)
3. Barbell Shrug: 3 sets of 5 reps (3x5)
4. Barbell Curl: 3 sets of 5 reps (3x5)

Friday:

1. Squat: 3 sets of 5 reps (3x5)
2. Romanian Deadlift: 3 sets of 5 reps (3x5)
3. Close Grip Bench Press: 3 sets of 5 reps (3x5)
4. Weighted Crunches: 3 sets of 15 reps (3x15)

I personally prefer the three days per week workout. Mentally, I find it easier to go all out on four exercises as opposed to six. I know I don't have to hold back any effort early in my workout so I can make it through six exercises. It is the routine that I am doing right now as of the writing of this book. But I now know that no matter how carefully I manage my poundage progressions, at some point, I am going to "hit the wall" and plateau. My progress will stagnate and it will be time to try something else to begin moving forward again. There will have to be another strategy to turn to in order to kickstart progression once more. The way to do this will be explained in the next chapter.

"Think about it this way. If you break a max by 5 pounds a month, that's 60 pounds a year. If you keep doing that, you're going to be a bad dude."

-Louie Simmons

Chapter 26

THE MOTIVATED AND FIT ADVANCED WORKOUT

(Advanced Progression Phase)

This phase is for men and women who:

1. Have completed *Progression Phase One* and progressed as far as they could in their first go around of the *Intermediate Progression Phase*.
2. May be coming back from an illness or minor injury that may have sidelined them for a few days or weeks and need a good "jump in" point.
3. Are over 50 years of age and don't feel they have the recovery ability to continually work at 85% or above intensity on their workouts without burnout.

The advanced trainee can't lift 90% to 100% of his or her 3x5 weight on any given exercise year-round. There has to be back off periods where the mind and body get a bit of a break and where the body can establish a "gaining momentum." What is easier? Running up a hill by starting your run at the base of the hill or giving yourself a running start on flat ground before you get to the base of the hill? Of course, a running start on flat ground will get you up the hill much easier.

This is a strategy that is used in the *Advanced Progression Phase*. It uses a plan based on poundage cycling.

Poundage cycling is a system that has been used by European lifters as far back as the pre-1950s. I first learned it from a strength coach back in the mid-1980s. His name was Barry Rubin. Barry simply had me apply poundage cycling to the bodybuilding routine that I was already using. Over a three-month period, my strength improved significantly and I put on eight pounds of muscle. I still utilize poundage cycling at least three to four months out of the year. However, I have tweaked the system over the years and have come up with my own version that I have found to be quite effective.

Poundage cycling is simply a way of building in a **back off** period where the training is not so hard. The "not so hard" weeks allow recovery from the near maximum training effort that preceded it. This system is about **nudging** the body into greater strength and increased muscle rather than **forcing** it. Similar to all of life, growth comes in cycles.

So how do you perform a poundage cycle? This can most easily be explained by taking your top 3x5 weight from the intermediate workout in each exercise and multiplying those numbers by .775, .85, .925, and one. These numbers will give you the weights to use for the first four weeks of the cycle.

For the sake of convenience, let's assume your maximum 3x5 weight on the barbell curl was 100 pounds. Your first four weeks of barbell curls break down this way:

Week 1: 100 lbs. x .775 (77.5%) = 77.5 lbs. x 3 x 5
Week 2: 100 lbs. x .85 (85%) = 85 lbs. x 3 x 5
Week 3: 100 lbs. x .925 (92.5%) = 92.5 lbs. 3 x 5
Week 4: 100 lbs. x 1 (100%) = 100 lbs. x 3 x 5

Stated another way, you will perform:
- 3 x 5 with 77.5 lbs. on barbell curls in week 1
- 3 x 5 with 85 lbs. on barbell curls in week 2
- 3 x 5 with 92.5 lbs. on barbell curls in week 3
- 3 x 5 with 100 lbs. on barbell curls in week 4

The first month of poundage cycling will give your body a nice recovery break. The first three weeks will be refreshing. The all-out effort that was given week after week in the Intermediate phase will make the first 3 weeks of your new poundage cycle feel like a walk in the park! There is a nice bonus in week number four; the weights used in week four on the 3 x 5 sets will seem somewhat lighter than those same weights did four weeks ago in the Intermediate workout. Starting at 77.5% of your top weights gives you the running start on flat ground to make it up the hill.

So, what do you do in month 2 of poundage cycling? I have learned that an increase of 2.5% of my previous top poundages was always challenging but usually attainable. Taking the previous example of the barbell curl once more, our next month of poundage cycling would like this with a 2.5% increase in mind:

- 100 lbs. x .025 (2.5%) = 2.5 lbs.
- 100 lbs. + 2.5 lbs. = 102.5 lbs.

Week 1: 102.5 lbs. x .775 = 80 lbs. x 3 x 5
Week 2: 102.5 lbs. x .85 = 87 lbs. x 3 x 5
Week 3: 102.5 lbs. x .925 = 95 lbs. x 3 x 5
Week 4: 102. 5 lbs. x 1 = 102.5 lbs. x 3 x 5

Once we determine our percentages, we have a couple of options. Using the fractional plates, as I suggested earlier, we can come very close to nailing every percentage weight that we derive from our poundage cycling formula. I know that many will not utilize the fractional plates. If the fractional plates are not used, we will have to either round up or round down some of our numbers. Thus, the barbell curl weights each week would look something like the following:

Week 1: 80 lbs. x 3 x 5
Week 2: 90 lbs. x 3 x 5
Week 3: 100 lbs. x 3 x 5
Week 4: 105 lbs. x 3 x 5

The above percentages were derived by rounding up the 3 x 5 maximum percentage from 102.5 lbs. to 105 lbs. Given a choice, I tend to round up when needed rather than rounding down.

While a 2.5% increase may not seem like much to some, it adds up over a 3 or 4 month period. To use a more dramatic example, let's take an exercise where more weight can be used, such as the bench press. Let's assume that you can bench press 225 lbs. for 3 x 5. If you increased your maximum 3 x 5 weight 2.5% per month over a 3 month period, that would mean you could perform 241 lbs. for 3 x 5 on the bench press.

Now, THAT IS PROGRESS! Also take into account that the vast majority of those in the gym lift the same weights for the same sets and reps day after day and month after month! Where is there any progression at all?

Making calculated, sensible poundage progression is a much better bet in terms of making gains in muscle and strength. So, don't laugh at just getting 2.5% stronger each month. Little bits of progress add up to huge chunks over time!

You can't just walk into the gym and randomly lift in hopes of getting a stronger and more muscular body. A goal without a plan is just a dream! When you are ready for the **Motivated and Fit Advanced Workout** give it a 3 to 4 month try and watch your body soar to new levels.

Using your top 3 x 5 rep poundages from the Inter-mediate phase, your first 2 months of poundage cycling will look something similar to the following routine. For the sake of simplicity, percentage poundages were rounded either up or down. Again, to precisely hit your percentages, break out your fractional plates.

I have provided some examples of the Poundage Cycle for Month 1 and Month 2 on the following pages.

*NOTE - Remember that the weights used in Weeks 1, 2, and 3 are determined by the weights you plan on lifting in Week 4; thus, it might be helpful to look at week 4 first before looking at Weeks 1, 2, and 3.

POUNDAGE CYCLE - MONTH 1

WEEK 1 – 77.5%

MON	Bench Press: 175 x 3 x 5	Bent Over Row: 115 x 3 x 5	Calf Raise: 235 x 3 x 15	Hanging Leg Raise: BW x 3 x 15
WED	Barbell Overhead Press: 105 x 3 x 5	Trap Bar Deadlift: 235 x 3 x 5	Barbell Shrug: 215 x 3 x 5	Barbell Curl: 80 x 3 x 5
FRI	Squat: 200 x 3 x 5	Romanian Dead Lift: 155 x 3 x 5	Close Grip Bench Press: 145 x 3 x 5	Weighted Crunches: 35 x 3 x 15

WEEK 2 – 85%

MON	Bench Press: 190 x 3 x 5	Bent Over Row: 130 x 3 x 5	Calf Raise: 260 x 3 x 15	Hanging Leg Raise: BW x 3 x 15
WED	Barbell Overhead Press: 115 x 3 x 5	Trap Bar Deadlift: 255 x 3 x 5	Barbell Shrug: 235 x 3 x 5	Barbell Curl: 85 x 3 x 5
FRI	Squat: 215 x 3 x 5	Romanian Dead Lift: 170 x 3 x 5	Close Grip Bench Press: 160 x 3 x 5	Weighted Crunches: 40 x 3 x 15

WEEK 3 – 92.5%

MON	Bench Press: 210 x 3 x 5	Bent Over Row: 140 x 3 x 5	Calf Raise: 280 x 3 x 5	Hanging Leg Raise: BW x 3 x 15
WED	Barbell Overhead Press: 125 x 3 x 5	Trap Bar Deadlift: 280 x 3 x 5	Barbell Shrug: 255 x 3 x 5	Barbell Curl: 95 x 3 x 5
FRI	Squat: 235 x 3 x 5	Romanian Dead Lift: 185 x 3 x 5	Close Grip Bench Press: 170 x 3 x 5	Weighted Crunches: 45 x 3 x 15

WEEK 4 – 100%

MON	Bench Press: 225 x 3 x 5	Bent Over Row: 150 x 3 x 5	Calf Raise: 300 x 3 x 15	Hanging Leg Raise: BW x 3 x 15
WED	Barbell Overhead Press: 135 x 3 x 5	Trap Bar Deadlift: 300 x 3 x 5	Barbell Shrug: 275 x 3 x 5	Barbell Curl: 100 x 3 x 5
FRI	Squat: 255 x 3 x 5	Romanian Dead Lift: 200 x 3 x 5	Close Grip Bench Press: 185 x 3 x 5	Weighted Crunches: 50 x 3 x 15

POUNDAGE CYCLE - MONTH 2
(with 2.5% poundage increase)

WEEK 1 – 77.5%

MON	Bench Press: 180 x 3 x 5	Bent Over Row: 120 x 3 x 5	Calf Raise: 240 x 3 x 15	Hanging Leg Raise: BW x 3 x 15
WED	Barbell Overhead Press: 110 x 3 x 5	Trap Bar Deadlift: 240 x 3 x 5	Barbell Shrug: 220 x 3 x 5	Barbell Curl: 80 x 3 x 5
FRI	Squat: 200 x 3 x 5	Romanian Dead Lift: 160 x 3 x 5	Close Grip Bench Press: 150 x 3 x 5	*Weighted Crunches: 40 x 3 x 15

*NOTE: The least you will be able to realistically increase on the weighted crunch with either a machine or free weights is 5 pounds. You will have to jump the weight up a little here, or stay with the weight used during the last poundage cycle and increase the reps. Another option would be to change to another exercise for the abs entirely if you wish to do so.

WEEK 2 – 85%

MON	Bench Press: 195 x 3 x 5	Bent Over Row: 130 x 3 x 5	Calf Raise: 265 x 3 x 15	Hanging Leg Raise: BW x 3 x 15
WED	Barbell Overhead Press: 120 x 3 x 5	Trap Bar Deadlift: 265 x 3 x 5	Barbell Shrug: 245 x 3 x 5	Barbell Curl: 90 x 3 x 5
FRI	Squat: 225 x 3 x 5	Romanian Dead Lift: 175 x 3 x 5	Close Grip Bench Press: 160 x 3 x 5	*Weighted Crunches: 45 x 3 x 15

WEEK 3 – 92.5%

MON	Bench Press: 215 x 3 x 5	Bent Over Row: 145 x 3 x 5	Calf Raise: 290 x 3 x 15	Hanging Leg Raise: BW x 3 x 15
WED	Barbell Overhead Press: 130 x 3 x 5	Trap Bar Deadlift: 290 x 3 x 5	Barbell Shrug: 265 x 3 x 5	Barbell Curl: 100 x 3 x 5
FRI	Squat: 245 x 3 x 5	Romanian Dead Lift: 190 x 3 x 5	Close Grip Bench Press: 175 x 3 x 5	*Weighted Crunches: 50 x 3 x 15

WEEK 4 – 100%

MON	Bench Press: 230 x 3 x 5	Bent Over Row: 155 x 3 x 5	Calf Raise: 310 x 3 x 15	Hanging Leg Raise: BW x 3 x 15
WED	Barbell Overhead Press: 140 x 3 x 5	Trap Bar Deadlift: 310 x 3 x 5	Barbell Shrug: 285 x 3 x 5	Barbell Curl: 105 x 3 x 5
FRI	Squat: 265 x 3 x 5	Romanian Dead Lift: 205 x 3 x 5	Close Grip Bench Press: 190 x 3 x 5	*Weighted Crunches: 55 x 3 x 15

As stated earlier, I like to perform poundage cycling for 3 or 4 consecutive months each year. For those who find recovery from workouts problematic, it might be THE PREDOMINANT WAY for you to train most of the year. The set and rep schemes presented (3x5) are definitely not the only ones that can be used. With a little bit of experimentation and self-testing in the gym, you can discover what your set and rep maximums are for a myriad of set/rep combinations. You can try 2 x 15, 3 x 10, 4 x 8, 3 x 3, or even something as seemingly crazy as 10 x 1(only if you a VERY advanced!). Single rep training will be explained in the next chapter.

> "As soon as a milestone is passed, it's significance fades, and the focus is shifted to some other marker down the road. No matter what you do or how satisfying it is in that beautiful moment in time, immediately you want more. You have to, if you want to find out how good you can be."
>
> -Glenn Pendlay

Chapter 27

SINGLE REP TRAINING

You only have to look at today's powerlifters and Olympic lifters to see the value of performing single rep training. Both of these types of lifters often carry enough muscle on their body to look almost "freakish." Powerlifters and Olympic lifters all use single rep lifts as a vital part of their programs. Most do sets of low reps along with five to ten sets of singles with 90 to 95% of their one rep max. Anyone who seeks the highest levels of strength development must admit that a man who can lift the heavier weight for one rep is considered stronger than the man who does more reps with a given weight, but with a lighter weight. Combine some single rep training on the big lifts in your workouts and watch your strength and muscle development soar!

First off, single rep training is for advanced trainees only! This means that if you are a male that can't bench press, squat, and deadlift 300/400/500 pounds respectively, save this program for later. Women need to hold off on this program until they hit the benchmarks of 150/225/300 pounds in these three lifts.

Secondly, there are just a few exercises that I feel lend themselves to single rep sets. They are the "big" exercises like squats, deadlifts, bench presses, barbell overhead presses, and power cleans. When utilizing single rep training, I usually do just one exercise per workout where single reps are performed. That exercise is always done first in my workouts. Let's use the barbell overhead press as our single rep exercise example. Someone who can perform a max single of 260 pounds in the barbell overhead press would use the following percentages, weights, and sets in the first workout of their program:

SET 1:
130 lbs. (50% of 1 rep max) x 10 reps (warm up set)

SET 2:
195 lbs. (75% of 1 rep max) x 5 reps (warm up set)

SET 3, 4, 5, 6, and 7:
242 lbs. (93% of 1 rep max for 5 sets) x 1 rep

SET 6, 7, and 8:
155 lbs. (60% of 1 rep max taken to near failure each set—this will put you somewhere in the 8-12 rep range on these 3 sets).

The next time you perform the barbell overhead press, you will add a 1 rep set to the workout, meaning that you will now be doing 6 sets of 1 rep sets with 242 pounds. Adding a set each workout will be your means of progression. Add a 1 rep set each workout until you are performing 10 sets of 1 rep sets with 242 pounds. (10 x 1 x 242 lbs.). After performing the 10 x 1 workout, rest 5 days and test for a new 1 rep max. Let's say it is now 275 pounds. You start a new cycle beginning with 5 sets of 1 rep, but now with a heavier weight. Repeat the same process as the first cycle. Some other important tips when doing single rep training are:

- Rest 4 minutes between 1 rep sets.
- Do no more than 3 to 4 more exercises for a maximum of 5 sets per exercise after performing your single rep exercise to prevent overtraining.

I like this particular routine because you get the strength/power building component from the 1 rep sets as well as the muscular hypertrophy component from the 60% weights for the 3 sets of 8-12 reps. A good routine with single rep training as the focal point looks like this:

MON	Bench Press: 1 x 10, 1 x 5, *5-10 x 1, 3 x 8-12	Bent Over Row: 5 x 5	Incline Dumbbell Curl 3 x 8	One Dumbbell Calf Raise: 3 x 15
WED	Barbell Overhead Press: 1 x 10, 1 x 5, *5-10 x 1, 3 x 8-12	Romanian Dead Lift: 5 x 5	Barbell Shrug: 5 x 5	Crunch Sit-Up: 3 x 15
FRI	Squats: 1 x 10, 1 x 5, *5-10 x 1, 3 x 8-12	Close Grip Bench Press: 5 x 5	Chip Up: 3 x 10	Seated Calf Raise: 3 x 15

This style of training is very tough; especially when you are getting closer to 10 x 1 on the big lifts in this routine. Feel free to change the exercises listed here. This is just a template. Remember to incorporate plenty of quality food and rest to maximize recovery. Now, hit the gym with determination and the resolve to get bigger and stronger than ever!

"A weak man is not as happy as that same man would be if he were strong."
-Mark Rippetoe

Chapter 28

1963
MR. AMERICA'S WORKOUT

The great bodybuilders of yesteryear did it differently. Their training tended to be much more abbreviated and efficient. This was the case for 1963 Mr. America Vern Weaver. He had incredible symmetry and a very good amount of muscle mass for that time period. His main off-season workout was the following:

MONDAY AND THURSDAY

1. Decline Bench Press: 6 x 6
2. Weighted Chin Ups: 6 x 6

TUESDAY AND FRIDAY

1. Bottom Position Squats in Power Rack: 6 x 6
2. High Pulls: 6 x 6

That's it. Weaver's sessions were completed in under an hour. Simplicity and efficiency at its best!

You don't have to live in the gym to make big muscle gains. You do need to have GOALS, A PLAN, INTENSITY, and CONSISTENCY! There are no magic lifting programs. Use the KISS principle (keep it simple, stupid) and get to work!

> "Stimulate, don't annihilate."
>
> -Lee Haney

Chapter 29

PRESSED FOR TIME?

(From my workout journal dated 11/30/18)

I could see that this week was going to be one in which I would be very pressed for time. I knew there would be no way that I would be able to get in my regular three workouts per week. You must sometimes change your training regimen a little for a week or two when time is scarce. Thus, I just finished my second of two workouts that I scheduled for myself this week. This is the routine I used:

MONDAY

Bench Press from Bottom Position in Power Rack:
5 x 5, 5 x 1

Squat from Bottom Position in Power Rack:
5 x 5, 5 x 1

FRIDAY

Barbell Overhead Press: 5 x 5, 5 x 1

Trap Bar Deadlift: 5 x 5, 5 x 1

It looks easy, but it's not! (especially the Monday routine with the bottom position Bench Press and

Squats). Most of the major muscle groups in the body get hit to varying degrees, and the natural testosterone production that these exercises generate is significant. Next week I will be back to my regular training routine where I work out on more days and perform more exercises with less sets per exercise. I enjoyed knowing that I only had two exercises to GO ALL-OUT ON, despite doing numerous sets of each. It really narrowed my mental focus. Keep the above routine in mind when you know you will only have a couple of days in which you can train in a particular week. Do what you have to do to STAY IN THE GAME!

"Working chest, delts, triceps, and biceps works approximately 10% of your overall lean body mass. Working hard on deadlifts (bent legged), trap bar, or sumo, and squatting (not necessarily at the same time) works more like 70% of your musculature at once and sends a strong message to your body to get better at growing now!"

-Wesley Silveira

Chapter 30

STAY ON YOUR FEET

The most productive weight training exercises are performed with barbells and dumbbells and not with machines or sitting on a bench. And the most growth producing exercises are done while **standing on your feet!** Old time pre-steroid era bodybuilders performed just about all of their exercises from a standing position and had enviable strength and physique development. Look up guys such as George Hackenschmidt and John Grimek. They had mind-blowing strength and development, and both were from the pre-World War II period, before the age of advanced exercise equipment and modern pharmaceuticals. Absolute studs! What exercises did they do?

Squats
Power Cleans
High Pulls
Barbell Bent Rows
Overhead Press
Snatches
Super-heavy one and two-handed dumbbell work
Deadlifts

"Far too many bodybuilders spend too much time exercising the smaller muscle groups such as the biceps at the expense of the larger muscle groups such as the thighs and then they wonder why it is that they never make gains in overall size and strength."

-Reg Park

Chapter 31

IF I COULD TURN BACK TIME

I often wish I could go back to when I started weight training and get a do-over. At 15 years of age, my training was good, but if I knew then what I know now, goals would have been reached MUCH sooner and more efficiently. There are several things I wish I could have told my 15-year-old self to do differently.

I would have told myself to focus on progressive poundage increases on the squat, deadlift, and bench press. If I had done so, I would have been as close to being as big and strong as I had ever dreamed of by 25 years of age. The overhead (military) press, bent rows, and heavy curls also would have received attention. Isolation exercises like the dumbbell fly, lateral raises, and leg extensions would have been added to my routines ONLY after I had achieved 300/400/500-pound maximums on the bench press, squat and dead-lift respectively. I would have chiseled the statue ONLY after I had a big rock to chisel from!

However, I cannot turn back time. My training mistakes have been valuable in that I can use them to advise others as to what NOT TO DO. One of my desires now is to reach as many young lifters as possible and help give them the start that I wish I could have had.

"Always remember this… there is only ONE recipe for strength. A secret recipe that was handed down from Sandow to John Grimek to Vasily Alexeev to Bill Kazmaier to me. Now I'm giving YOU that magic recipe… hard work plus proper nutrition plus time equals strong."

-Steve Pulcinella

Chapter 32

THE CASE FOR USING ISOLATION EXERCISES

By now, all of you realize that my training philosophy is based on the use of basic, multi-joint compound free weight exercises and little else. These exercises include squats, deadlifts, power cleans, bench presses, military presses, etc. The basic exercises work more than one muscle at a time and give you more bang for the buck.

Isolation exercises work one muscle group at the exclusion of others. Isolation movements have an exclusive focus on a specific body part being worked without involving any other muscle groups. Examples of isolation exercises are lateral raises for the deltoids, dumbbell flyes for the chest, and leg extensions for the thighs. I don't consider isolation exercises as an important part of my training due to the fact that they are just not an economical choice as far as exercise selection is concerned.

Does this mean I don't ever use isolation exercises? No. There are times when they are part of my routine. There are times when isolation movements are valuable. A number of situations exist where isolation exercises can be very beneficial. The following is a list of situations where the use of isolation exercises make sense:

WHEN HEAVY WEIGHTS BEGIN TO BOTHER YOUR JOINTS OR CAUSE INJURY

After months of lifting heavy iron, the joints could get sore. For example, my shoulder joints became irritated a few months ago. I dropped the heavy standing military presses for my shoulder work. I replaced my shoulder work with 3 shoulder isolation exercises: front cable raises, side lateral raises, and bent lateral raises. This gave my shoulders a break from the heavy pounding. I utilized reps in the 8-12 range to maintain my size. After about a month, I was able to return to my heavy military pressing with no pain. In another case, my lower back was feeling like it was on the verge of injury. It became painful to squat, deadlift, or leg press. After about 3 weeks of replacing the heavy exercises with leg extensions, sissy squats, and leg curls (along with 3 chiropractic adjustments), I was able to return to the type of lifting I love once again.

BODYBUILDING COMPETITIONS

If you are a competing bodybuilder or have aspirations to compete AFTER YOU HAVE ALREADY BUILT CONSIDERABLE SIZE, isolation movements will be needed. Those of us whose competitive days are over (like yours truly) and those who have no aspirations to ever compete need not make much consideration of isolation exercises. The basics will get you as big and strong as you will ever want to be. However, isolation exercises will give the competitive bodybuilder the ability to round out and perfect the appearance of particular muscles when on stage.

In competitive bodybuilding, the margin of error between winning and losing is razor thin. Someone having an advantage as small as better rear deltoid development or a little bit more sweep on the quadriceps than the next guy is often the difference between a 1st and 2nd place trophy.

VARIETY AND NEW GROWTH STIMULUS

There are times for many of us when training just is not that fun anymore. Often what is needed is a layoff from training to recharge your batteries. At other times, a radical change in training to break up what you perceive as monotony is required. A month of more traditional bodybuilding training where half of your exercises are isolation moves might fit the bill. More training enthusiasm is often the result of a change like this.

The utilization of isolation movements combined with basic compound movements in a bodybuilding routine can cause a stimulus to the body that can "shock" it into more growth. Combining isolation exercises with multi joint exercises will considerably increase your training volume. If overdone, this can quickly result in overtraining for the natural lifter. About a month to six weeks of this type of routine is recommended before returning to your regular style of training revolving around the basics.

Isolation exercises can be very useful when used under the right circumstances. Remember that the big basic movements are what truly builds muscle and might. But isolation exercises can be handy gadgets to have in your toolbox.

"You've got to block out all distractions when you train. Your focus has to be 100% into the rep. You've got to get into a zone. You know you're in the zone when guys in the gym look you in the eye and then quickly turn away 'cause they see the fire. You've got to be all business."

-Mike Matarazzo

Chapter 33

PRE-EXHAUST TRAINING

Pre-exhaustion training became widely known in the late 1970's and 1980's when promoted by legendary pro bodybuilders such as Mike and Ray Mentzer, Casey Viator, and exercise pioneer Arthur Jones (who invented the original Nautilus machines). Pre-exhaustion training first involves performing an isolation movement (like lateral raises for the deltoids) immediately followed by a multi-joint compound movement (like overhead dumbbell presses for the deltoids). No rest is taken between executing the isolation movement and the multi joint compound movement. When no rest is taken between two or more exercises, it is called a superset.

Why do pre-exhaust supersets work? It eliminates weak links that do not allow targeted muscles to get maximally stimulated when performing compound multi-joint movements like the overhead dumbbell press. For example, when someone is attempting to work their deltoids by pressing a weight overhead, two muscles are actually being used to accomplish this: the deltoids AND the smaller tricep muscle. Many individuals will incur muscular failure in the triceps first before the muscles of the deltoids can be maximally stimulated. However, if an exercise that uses no other muscles BUT the deltoids is used FIRST (like lateral raises), the deltoids will be hit hard before the next exercise (the overhead dumbbell press.) The deltoids will now become the muscle that fails first during the overhead dumbbell press. The triceps will be fresh and will be able to assist the deltoids into much greater fatigue. The deltoids will now reach muscular failure before the triceps, thus eliminating the triceps as the weak link.

The following is a pre-exhaust routine that I performed with former NPC Nationals Middleweight 3rd place finisher Lionel Gaubert in 1983. In retrospect, I had not yet built enough size and strength at this time to get the maximum benefit from pre-exhaust. Nonetheless, I learned how to perform pre-exhaust in the correct manner. This would prove to be valuable in the years to come (about ages 27-37).

MONDAY and THURSDAY
(chest, deltoids, triceps, and calves)

Chest
Dumbbell fly supersetted with bench press, 2 x 8-10

Deltoids
Lateral raises supersetted with overhead
dumbbell press, 2 x 8-10

Triceps
Tricep pushdown supersetted with dips, 2 x 8-10

Calves
Standing calf raises supersetted with seated calf raises,
2 x 8-12

TUESDAY and FRIDAY:
(back, biceps, thighs, hamstrings, and abs)

Back
Dumbbell pullover supersetted with lat pulldowns,
2 x 8-10

Biceps
Incline dumbbell curl supersetted with barbell curls,
2 x 8-10

Thighs
Leg extensions supersetted with leg press, 2 x 8-10

Hamstrings
Prone leg curls supersetted with Romanian deadlifts,
2 x 8-10

Note:
We called Romanian deadlifts "stiff legged deadlifts" at the time.

Abs
Hanging leg raises supersetted with crunches,
2 x 15-20

I honestly have not performed pre-exhaust since about 2003. Then, it was just performed as a break from the abbreviated, basic training style that I have utilized since 1993. I found that it was easy for me to overtrain using pre-exhaust once I approached age 40. However, I did make significant gains with it when I mixed it in here and there. If you need a little change of pace in your training, pre-exhaustion is definitely worth a try.

"Even though I realized I had more than average genetics to build strength and muscle, I still trained in the most grueling manner possible."

-Casey Viator

Chapter 34

3 DAYS PER WEEK WHOLE BODY VARIETY ROUTINE

Here is one of my favorite beginner 3 days per week whole body routines. I've used this one from time to time even after several decades of training. While I'm calling it a beginner routine, it can be used by advanced lifters who may need a break from higher volume training.

MONDAY:
- Leg Press 3 x 8-12
- Romanian Deadlift 3 x 8-12
- Lat Pulldown 3 x 8-12
- Bench Press 3 x 8-12
- Overhead Barbell Press 2 x 8-12
- Incline Dumbbell Curl 2 x 8-12
- Seated Dumbbell French Press 2 x 8-12
- Standing Calf Raise 2 x 8-12

WEDNESDAY:
- Squat 3 x 8-12
- One Arm Dumbbell Row 3 x 8-12
- Dips 3 x 8-12
- Side Lateral Raise 2 x 8-12

- Barbell Curl 2 x 8-12
- Lying EZ Bar Tricep Extension 2 x 8-12
- Calf Press 2 x 15
- Ab Crunch 2 x 15

FRIDAY:
- Trap Bar Deadlift 3 x 8-12
- Bent Over Barbell Row 3 x 8-12
- Incline Barbell Press 3 x 8-12
- Close Grip Bench Press 2 x 8-12
- Dumbbell Front Raise 2 x 8-12
- Bent Over Lateral Raise 2 x 8-12
- Seated Calf Raise 2 x 15
- Back Extension 2 x 15

"Health is a divine gift, and the care of the body is a sacred duty, to neglect which is a sin."

-Eugen Sandow

Chapter 35

DO YOU REALLY NEED THE PUMP?

It is a fallacy that you must get the "pump" during workouts for muscle growth. If you can move more weight in the close grip bench press and the curl than you did three months ago, size will increase as well.

Each week, my arm routine is made up of three sets of close grip bench press and three sets of curls. I usually only do five or six reps per exercise. I never get a blood gorging pump anywhere, just a slight increase in size from a little more blood getting to a particular body part. But I work hard. And despite a very low volume of work, I still sport arms that are over 18 inches cold and get up to 19 inches with just a few sets on a couple of arm exercises. Work hard on poundage progression, and the size will follow. Don't worry so much about the pump.

> "Your body, despite the science that says "X number of reps is better for this, Y for that" will get stronger if it is overloaded."
> -Dr. Ken Leistner

Chapter 36

FOCUS ON THE TASK AT HAND

When you get to the gym, you have to put everything else that has happened to you that day and any negative things going on in your life behind you! You must focus on the task at hand. Do not worry about the test you have next week, the presentation you have to give on Friday, or the girlfriend that just dumped you.

The gym is a place where you must focus on what you are doing. You must get done what you have to do without giving thought to anything else. I refer to the gym as my "sanctuary" or my favorite "getaway." When you walk into the gym, you must have the attitude that you have a job to do, and you will work with an uncluttered mind and controlled ferocity! In other words, get your head right and UNLEASH YOUR INNER BEAST!

> "When your drive is moving your purpose, focus must hold the wheels else you might miss the way. And do you know what that means? Avoid crash! Stay focused!"
> - Israelmore Ayivor

Chapter 37

THOSE STUBBORN CALVES

Calves are a difficult body part for many people to develop. There are many theories as to why. One of them is the fact that the muscles of the calf are predominantly made up of type 1 (aka slow twitch) muscle fibers. Slow twitch muscles have less hypertrophy potential than type 2 (fast twitch) muscle fibers. Thus, a lot of individuals feel that this causes the calves to be such a stubborn muscle to develop. Another theory is that there are less androgen receptors in the body the further you get away from the head/shoulder area. This would mean that the calves would have less androgen receptors than any other body part. By comparison, there are more androgen receptors in the neck and trapezius, with the number of androgen receptors decreasing as you move down the body.

The standing calf raise is considered the basic exercise for calf development. It works the two headed muscle of the calf called the gastrocnemius. The gastrocnemius is worked most efficiently with the knees straight or with just a slight bit of knee bend. Developing the gastrocnemius is a very important part of the equation in developing impressive calves. However, for full calf development you need to perform the seated calf raise. This isolates the soleus, the part of the calf that lies below the two heads of the gastrocnemius. With the knee bent at 90°, the soleus is activated in an isolatory manner, with the activation of the gastrocnemius pretty much eliminated. This ensures that the underlying soleus muscle gets hit HARD. As the calf is a three headed muscle, it makes sense that they will become bigger when all three heads are stimulated effectively. Since the soleus lies beneath the gastrocnemius, development of the soleus will push out the gastrocnemius, resulting in more overall size, circumference, and shape to the calf.

An important point when training the calves is to pause one second at the bottom of each rep and one second at the top of each rep. Pausing at the bottom of the rep keeps you from rebounding or bouncing to the top position and ensures that you use muscle strength only. Pausing at the top of the rep allows for a great peak contraction.

"Too many people leave the 'minor' body parts off. Areas like calves, abdominals, and trapezius muscles are often throw in body parts for a lot of folks. Proper volume, intensity and frequency of training these areas are often neglected. Remember, IF YOU WANT TO COMPETE, YOU MUST BE COMPLETE."

-Joel Lucky

Chapter 38

SO, WHO HAS WORKED LEGS THIS WEEK?

I was recently looking at a college photo of a father of a fairly well-known athlete. He had an impressive upper body for a college guy, but it was obvious that he liked to skip leg day! The poor guy had legs like a chicken. I am sometimes asked, "How do you get big arms?" I will answer, "The best way to get big arms is from hard, heavy squats!" Always getting a confused look, I go on to explain the hormonal response the body receives from intense leg work. Working legs is the **key** to putting on mounds of muscle throughout your entire body. A house built on a weak foundation will not stand. Powerful legs are your foundation. SO STOP SKIPPING LEG DAY AND GO DO SOME SQUATS!

Don't be the lifter who has the upper body of Hercules and the legs of Pee Wee Herman. Work on your entire body so your symmetry flows and you look complete. Don't leave out any body parts because you don't find them comfortable or fun to train. You've got to hit everything! When you look at classic physique stars such as Steve Reeves, Reg Park, Linda Murray, and Cory Everson, you will see that no body part sticks out over another. You can tell by looking at their bodies that they had no favorite body parts to train, but they were, instead, mindful of training their entire body as a unit. You know what you have to do to have a physique that turns heads, so go do it!

"No one can afford to neglect any of these groups. All, in fact, should be equally developed, those which are naturally weaker to greater extent than the others, until all are equally strong, when the object in view should be that of EQUAL all-around development."

-George Hackenschmidt (1908)

Chapter 39

THE ARMS RACE

When it comes to building your arms, more is not necessarily better. My very first bodybuilding mentor was a gentleman named Lionel Gaubert. He was Mr. Louisiana, Mr. Greater Gulf States, and took third place in the NPC Nationals twice. His brother James Gaubert was Mr. Universe. I was fortunate enough to be a training partner of Lionel's as a senior in high school. We trained hard! Lionel used high-intensity and low-volume in all of his workouts. A typical arm workout for us looked like this:

1. Barbell Curl 3 x 8-10
2. Incline Dumbbell Curl 3 x 8-10
3. Overhead Dumbbell Extension 3 x 8-10
4. Tricep Pushdown 3 x 8-10

Simple and effective. We went to failure on every set. (Looking back, I realized that I was overtraining as a natural bodybuilding teenager). However, the point is that if a national level bodybuilder only needed six sets to train his biceps and triceps, it is probably more than you will ever need either! As a 54-year-old natural lifter (I don't call myself a bodybuilder any more), I have to be very careful to keep a volume of exercise that will keep me from overtraining.

"Nothing comes easy, but as long as you're breathing, you're always one breath away from making your dreams a reality. Make every breath count."

-Kai Greene

Chapter 40

5 REASONS WHY WOMEN NEED TO LIFT WEIGHTS

Lifting weights for women is every bit as important as it is for men. Perhaps more so. The days of simply attending an aerobics class or cycling class and calling it your fitness program are over. Lifting weights will do more for women than any other type of exercise. Simply put, if a woman desires to become her healthiest, sexiest and most fit, she will choose to pump iron. The reasons for a woman to have a strong weight training program are numerous:

1.
LIFTNG WEIGHTS BURNS FAT
LIKE MARSHMALLOWS IN A FIRE

When lifting weights is put head to head against cardio exercise, lifting comes out on top in terms of calorie burn. Lifting weights burns calories both during and after exercise. After a tough weight workout, your body continues to use oxygen as the hours pass by. This is called excess post-exercise oxygen consumption (EPOC). In this process, a woman's body uses more oxygen, thus requiring more caloric expenditure and an increase in metabolism.

2.
THE MORE MUSCLE YOU HAVE,
THE MORE FAT YOU BURN

As a woman's lean muscle mass and strength increases, the body is able to more efficiently use calories. With more muscle, more calories are burned at rest. With each pound of muscle gained, a woman's body becomes more and more of a fat burning machine. Gaining muscle is a major component in losing fat.

3.
WEIGHT TRAINING
STRENGTHENS BONES

Weight training builds your bones, not just your muscles. For example, when you perform a squat, the muscles of the thigh will tug on the femur. The femur's bone cells react to this by creating new bone cells. Thus, bones become denser and stronger. Women have more of a propensity to be affected by osteoporosis. Weight training will help head off osteoporosis at the pass by creating more bone density and strength. This fact alone is a huge reason for any woman to begin weight training.

4.
LIFTING WEIGHTS
GIVES A WOMAN CURVES

All women want that sexy curve to their backside. Sure, tell me you don't—to quote Austin Powers, "Rrrriight." Weights can give a woman that much desired hour glass look. Wider shoulders, a smaller waist and curvy hips will give you a silhouette that will make your visually inspired man even crazier about you. (And don't kid yourself, all men are visually inspired.) Most importantly, the changes in appearance that pumping iron will give you will result in a feeling of accomplishment that is hard to top.

5.
LIFTING WEIGHTS
LOWERS STRESS LEVELS

Women are under more stress now than at any other time in our history. To borrow from a 1970's TV commercial, most women now are expected to "bring home the bacon, fry it up in a pan, and never let you forget you're a man." It is almost an expectancy in American society that a woman has to be a significant income provider, mother to their children, and a wife that meets the needs of a large percentage of husbands! Weight training is a great way for a woman to manage stress. The brain's feel-good transmitters and endorphins are produced when that stimulating workout is performed after a stressful day.

> "It's not weird to look at yourself in the mirror at the gym—that's why they are there! You have to make sure that you are doing things right."
>
> -Allison Sweeney

Chapter 41

WHEN SHOULD MY CHILD BEGIN STRENGTH TRAINING?

According to the American Academy of Pediatrics, a child can begin strength training as soon as 7 or 8 years of age. However, strength training at this age should be done only under the following conditions:

1. Get your child a check-up first.

2. Keep the weights light with higher repetitions (12-15).

3. Have an extreme focus on form and technique.

4. Keep volume and intensity at a low level to keep possible injuries to an absolute minimum.

5. Focus on free weights over machines, as machines are designed for longer limbs.

Make sure you are training your child for strength, not weightlifting or powerlifting. The latter two are competitive endeavors that kids need to at least be in their teens to attempt. Explain to your child that gaining muscle size is something that can take place after adolescence. Building muscle mass can be undertaken once physical and skeletal maturity have been attained.

The key goals for the young strength trainee should be the following:

1. Increase the strength of young bones.

2. Attain a healthy body weight.

3. Promoting healthy blood pressure and cholesterol levels.

4. Improve confidence and self-esteem.

"Children are not things to be molded, but are people to be unfolded."

-Jess Lair

Chapter 42

WARRIORS VS. WORRIERS

Do not be the person that worries about selecting the "perfect routine" and procrastinates about getting into the gym until you "do your research." If you really want to exercise, pick out a few basic exercises to utilize, lift hard, find a few modes of cardio to perform 3 times per week and BE A WARRIOR! Get after it!

Don't be the person that says, "I could have accomplished so much more with my life if I had actually tried something instead of being a spectator, ponderer, and procrastinator." Most of us will have some regrets, but the individual who takes consistent action will make sure that the number of them will be few! Don't spend time thinking about "HOW" you are going to train, just use the "Keep It Simple, Stupid" (KISS) principle, TAKE MASSIVE ACTION and go work out!

> "When you promise yourself something, make a commitment, you can't give up. Because when you're in the gym, you have to fulfill the promise you made to yourself. The people who can self-motivate, in any field, are usually the ones who win regardless of talent."
>
> -Tom Platz

Chapter 43

COMMON SENSE EXERCISE SELECTION

As time passes, especially at about age 40 and beyond, little injuries incurred in your training career show up. Joint pain, injury-like muscle pain, etc. start to bother you, especially on particular exercises. The name of the game is STAYING POWER. This means training for as long and as injury-free as possible. You may have to ELIMINATE some of your favorite exercises if they cause any type of pain before it becomes an injury. I don't care if it is Arnold's favorite exercise; if it does not feel right, DON'T DO IT! Replace the exercise with something that works the same muscle(s) and avoid any possible injuries!

> "A HARSH REALITY: You will not be able to train forever. Eventually, we all get to a point where we will not be able to apply our dedication and determination to anything, let alone training, diet, and recovery from workouts. SO, MAKE THE ABSOLUTE MOST OF YOUR TRAINING TODAY!"
>
> -Joel Lucky

Chapter 44

HOW TO PRODUCE TESTOSTERONE NATURALLY

EAT ENOUGH FAT

Eat .5 grams of fat per pound of body weight daily. Thus, if you weigh 200 pounds, you would eat 100 grams of fat a day. Don't eat more fat than this! The idea is to eat enough to put your body in an anabolic environment to gain muscle, not bodyfat.

AVOID OVERTRAINING

Be careful to not spend too much time in the gym pumping iron. Overtraining can lower your testosterone levels and put the brakes on mass building. Make use of abbreviated routines on basic exercises. There is no reason to be in the gym more than 90 minutes no matter what your genetics or perceived training tolerance might be.

LIMIT YOUR CARDIO

When attempting to maximize testosterone production, spend only 20 to 30 minutes three times per week on cardio. Too much cardio will decease your ability to produce max levels of testosterone naturally.

UTILIZE NATURAL
TESTOSTERONE BOOSTERS

Supplements such as Ashwagandha, Zinc, and Vitamin D have been very helpful to many lifters at naturally increasing testosterone levels.

FIND WAYS TO ELIMINATE STRESS

Stress can activate the release of cortisol, which can severely limit the recovery process that is needed for growth and repair. Testosterone can be significantly lowered in times of stress. Deep breathing, meditation, visualization, prayer, and music therapy are just a few ways to calm the waters of your soul.

FOCUS ON THE BIG EXERCISES

Squats and deadlifts are the key exercises to naturally increasing testosterone. They are the two most anabolic enhancing exercises that exist. Other exercises that work well are power cleans, overhead presses and bench presses. The key is utilizing exercises that work multiple muscle groups at one time with heavy weights and intense effort.

"If you look good, are in good health, and feel good about yourself, then you'll be more productive at work, you will be happier in your relationships with your friends and family, and consequently, you will be a more productive, contributing member to society, making the world a better place for all."

-Lee Labrada

Chapter 45

DON'T BE OVERLY DOGMATIC IN YOUR TRAINING PHILOSOPHY

I'm an old-school lifter. As a rule, my training revolves around 8 or 10 multi-joint basic exercises. I utilize free weights and ground based (feet on the ground) exercises for the vast majority of my exercise selections.

In the quest for complete development, you can't ignore science. For instance, some muscles respond well to the peak contraction principle. Triceps are one of these muscles. I like close grip bench presses as much as anyone and they are often in my routines, but they offer little in the way of peak contraction. I came across a dip machine that was effectively a tricep push down that allowed me to use more weight than the pushdown—and offer very nice peak contraction at the end of the movement. Some traditionalists resist the use of machines on anything other than a lat pull-down.

You have to open your mind, sometimes in spite of what you have been taught, to attain your best potential for physical development. REMAIN OPEN TO ANYTHING THAT CAN MAKE YOU BETTER!

"Man's proper stature is not one of mediocrity, failure, frustration, or defeat, but one of achievement, strength, and mobility. In short, man can and ought to be a hero.

- Mike Mentzer

Chapter 46

HOW MUCH CARDIO SHOULD I DO?

The Department of Health and Human Services recommends at least 150 minutes of moderate aerobic activity a week or 75 minutes of vigorous aerobic activity a week. A combination of moderate and vigorous activity works also.

Should this really be the correct cardio guideline for everyone, though? In my experience as a long-time personal trainer and competitive bodybuilder, I would say NO. The amount of cardio you need to perform depends on your goal. The above cardio guidelines are on the money if your goal is primarily general fitness without the goal of attaining considerable muscle mass. Add in 2-3 basic weight training sessions a week to the above cardio recommendation and you will have a well-rounded exercise program.

HOWEVER, if muscle mass and strength is your primary goal, you will have to scale back this amount of cardio a good bit. Why? Because this amount of cardio can make negative inroads on your recovery ability when trying to gain significant muscle. Muscle fibers are actually torn down while lifting weights; getting sufficient rest and recovery between workouts allows the muscle fibers to heal, build, and get stronger. If you are doing 5 moderate intensity cardio sessions of 30 minutes per session or 75 minutes per week of high intensity cardio training, you simply won't be maximizing your ability to build muscle.

Cardio is a much-needed component for anyone. For someone attempting to gain maximum muscle and strength, I recommend 3 moderate intensity cardio sessions a week for a duration of 30 minutes each OR high intensity cardio (such as Tabata) 3 times a week for a maximum of 20 minutes a session. This will provide the health benefits to the heart and lungs without sacrificing much in the way of muscle gain.

"Personalize your exercise program to exactly fit your individual goals and available time. One size does not fit all when it comes to creating the body you desire."

-Joel Lucky

Chapter 47

THE LOW INTENSITY STEADY STATE CARDIO PROGRAM (LISS)

Low Intensity Steady State Cardio (LISS) is how I perform the vast majority of my cardiovascular exercise. It helps me keep unwanted fat off when I'm in a mass building phase and allows me to burn fat when I'm in a fat burning phase for increased definition. Low Intensity Steady State Cardio (LISS) is simply the most common style of cardio that you see in gyms across the world. It is simple, proven, and effective. LISS consists of a cardio workout that is a continuous, steady effort; as opposed to interval cardio where you vary your energy output at various intensities throughout your workout. With LISS, you will simply sustain a fixed intensity (post warm up) throughout the entire workout.

LISS not only helps you get lean and stay lean, but it also increases endurance and contributes greatly to heart health. It is also a great endorphin producer, which helps elevate mood. LISS has also been proven to defend against insulin resistance by increasing insulin sensitivity.

LISS program types are varied and numerous. Stair climbing machines, stationary bikes, treadmills, or elliptical machines are all great ways to utilize LISS in the gym. For those that prefer the outdoors—jogging, walking, or biking are all common ways of performing LISS.

If you are a beginner, take it easy starting out. Begin with 15 minutes per session and gradually increase your LISS training 20 or 25 minutes, eventually working your way up to 30 to 45 minute sessions. Perform LISS workouts 3-6 times per week. One must be careful to ensure that they create enough intensity to get the job done. Between 65% and 85% of your maximum heart rate will do. A good rule of thumb is if you can easily have a conversation with someone working out next to you, you probably need to increase your workout intensity.

"Cardio is a nice way to start in the morning, man. Whether you sit on the bike for half an hour or throw on two jumpers and just sweat, it's good to get up, get the body active, put on your headphones, and just pedal away."
-Anthony Joshua

Chapter 48

HOW TO DETERMINE TARGET HEART RATE FOR LOW INTENSITY STEADY STATE CARDIO (LISS)

The first step in determining a prescription for cardio-vascular exercise is determining target heart rate. This is achieved by simply subtracting your age from 220. For example, let's say you are 45 years old. Your maximum heart rate would be 175 beats per minute (bpm).

220-45= 175 bpm (maximum heart rate)

With your maximum heart rate (175 bpm), you can now calculate what your target heart rate should be. You will be using a percentage of your maximum heart rate to determine what your exercising heart rate would be. Most people will be able to exercise somewhere between 65% and 85% of your maximum heart rate. Experience with my personal training clients has shown that this is a good cardio range for general health purposes and fat loss. In the above example, the formula for calculating target heart rate for a 45-year-old would be as follows:

220-45 (age) x .65 or .85

We will use both 65% and 85% to give us a target heart rate range to work with. It will be easier to hit between these numbers than hitting an exact number. Thus, finding the range for a 45-year-old would look like this:

220-45= 175 x .65 = 113.75
220-45= 175 x .85 = 148.5

BINGO! Our 45-year-old needs their cardiovascular exercise to place them somewhere between 114 and 149 bpm. A typical cardio session should land somewhere between these two numbers (75%). A target heart rate of approximately 131 is where your heart rate should be for the majority of your work out. If you are just beginning cardiovascular exercise, you could start out at 65% of your maximum heart rate or even lower. Just start at whatever point you can, be consistent with your exercise regimen, and get fit!

"Don't count the days; make the days count."
-Muhammad Ali

Chapter 49

H.I.I.T. ME BABY
ONE MORE TIME

We all have busy lives. Some stretches of time are much busier than others. Recently, I have had to juggle writing a book, working a full-time job, and being a father of 2 teenage boys and husband to my beautiful wife—all while trying to stay in shape! Effective time management skills must be utilized when life gets hectic.

High Intensity Interval Training (HIIT) is a very good option when you have limited time for your workouts. Twenty minutes maximum of HIIT will get the job done when pressed for time. As previously stated, I have a preference for Low Intensity Steady State Cardio (LISS). But sometimes you have to do what you have to do!

HIIT has several benefits. The short bursts of all out exercise used when performing HIIT can rev up your metabolism for up to 24 hours after you have completed the exercise session. This means you can actually burn calories the next day by sitting on the couch! Not a bad deal. Another big benefit of HIIT is the elevation of human growth hormone (HGH) that occurs when performing this type of fat burning exercise. HGH is a chemical that builds muscle and melts fat away in the body. HGH production slows down as we age, but it can be boosted as we get older by stimulating HGH production with this type of exercise.

So, what version of HIIT do I recommend? I like to use what is called TABATA. TABATA training comes from Japan. Japanese scientist Dr. Izumi Tabata and a team of researchers from the National Institute of Fitness and Sports in Tokyo created this style of cardiovascular training.

My TABATA exercise program is as follows:

- All out sprinting on the treadmill, battle rope work, burpees, rowing machine, etc. done for 20 seconds.

- Rest for 10 seconds between each exercise.

- Complete 40 rounds of the 20 second exercise intervals.

Starting out, you will be better off doing a total of 4 minutes, which would be 8 rounds of all out 20 second exercise intervals. If you are new to this type of training, break into it very slowly. Every fourth workout, add a couple of rounds until you reach the maximum recommended 40 rounds of TABATA training.

My workout will look something like the following: I will start off with 20 seconds of all-out effort on the rowing machine and rest 10 seconds. I will then move to 20 seconds of wave patterns using the battle ropes. After another 10 second rest, I will perform 20 seconds of burpees. The final exercise of the series could be 20 seconds of treadmill sprints.

CONSIDERATIONS FOR USING TABATA:

1. Use TABATA music that works as a timer for your 20 second exercise/10 second rest intervals. I simply use my cell phone and go to YouTube to find this. The music will have added to it a voice that will tell you when to start the 20 second exercise interval as well as a 5 second countdown before giving you the signal to take your 10 second rest. You will also get a 5 second countdown to lead you into the next 20 second exercise interval.

2. Perform TABATA on days that you do not perform weight training. It is a very intense exercise method that could quickly lead to overtraining if performed on the same day as the weights.

3. If you are using weights, perform TABATA no more than 3 days per week. Between weight training and TABATA, this will give you 5 or 6 intense exercise bouts a week, which is plenty of work over the course of the week.

4. If you are over 40 years of age, consider performing TABATA only 2 days per week. Also consider possibly doing the least amount of 20 second exercise intervals to get the job done. Many find that 4 to 8 total minutes of TABATA is all they need to get results. As we get older and begin to have less efficient recovery abilities,

we find that less is sometimes more. When life is hectic, consider this style of cardiovascular training. TABATA is very time efficient and a great way to fit in cardio exercise when your time is scarce.

"Strength does not come from physical capacity. It comes from indomitable will."
-Ghandi

Chapter 50

LOSE FAT WITH THIS SIMPLE MEAL PLAN

Finding a diet that will work to lose fat does not have to be a complicated matter. Apply the following simple principles and you will not have to count calories, carbohydrates, or fat grams. You will lose fat and maintain lean body mass, with no big fuss, hassle, or calculations.

First, think of dividing your food plate into thirds. On one third of your plate, you will have a lean protein source such as a chicken breast, fish, or beef. On another third of your plate, you will have a complex carbohydrate such as brown rice, whole grain pasta, or sweet potato. The final third of the plate will consist of a fibrous carbohydrate such as broccoli, squash, or cauliflower. For most men, a plate which is 8 inches in diameter will work; for most women, a 6-inch diameter plate will do. You will eat three meals like this per day along with 16 oz of water per meal.

Another two or three meals can be taken in the form of a low-sugar protein drink or protein bar. A day of eating like this will look something like the following:

9 A.M.	Myoplex protein drink
12 P.M.	1 chicken breast, brown rice, green beans, water
3 P.M.	Quest protein bar, water
6 P.M.	Lean cut of steak, whole grain pasta, cauliflower, water
9 P.M.	Baked fish, sweet potato, broccoli, water

Stick to this basic plan for 60 days and watch what happens to your body! Along with some weight training and cardiovascular exercise, this simple but effective eating style will work wonders.

"It's simple. If it jiggles, it's fat."
-Arnold Schwarzenegger

Chapter 51

LOW GLYCEMIC INDEX CARBS: THE BETTER CARB CHOICE

The glycemic index is a system assigning a number to carbohydrate foods based on how much each food increases blood sugar. Low glycemic index carbohydrates break down more slowly, which allows the release of glucose more gradually into the blood stream. Slower glucose release into the bloodstream has multiple benefits such as:

- Improved appetite control
- Increasing sensitivity to insulin
- Decreasing the risk of heart disease
- Improving diabetes control
- Reducing blood cholesterol levels; decreasing and controlling weight
- Minimizing energy crashes
- Helping prolong physical endurance

Examples of low GI carbs (YES CARBS) include:

- Sweet potatoes
- Yams
- Brown rice
- Whole grain pasta

Examples of high GI carbs (NO-NO CARBS) include:

- White bread
- Corn
- Potatoes
- Regular pasta

As mentioned earlier, each carbohydrate food has a GI value. For the most part, the number is based on how much a food item raises blood glucose levels compared to how much pure glucose raises blood glucose. Glycemic index values are basically divided into 3 categories:

Low GI:	**1-55**
Medium GI:	**56-69**
High GI:	**70 and above**

When choosing which carbohydrate foods you eat, try to eat predominately low and medium GI carbs. Whether the goal is to stay healthy, lose fat, or gain lean muscle, they are the way to go!

"Eat for nutrition and food value. Emphasize natural foods, avoid processed foods, and eliminate junk entirely."

-Vince Gironda

Chapter 52

INTERMITTENT FASTING

Intermittent Fasting (IF) is a nutrition plan that I have used with excellent results. In the summer of 2018, I was looking to lower my bodyfat levels while maintaining my muscle mass. Intermittent fasting definitely got the job done.

So, what is IF? Basically, you fast for 16 hours a day and only allow yourself to eat within an 8-hour window during a 24-hour period. The only thing permitted during fasting hours is water or black coffee. (Note: There are many versions of IF—this is just one of the basic versions and one that I have personally utilized.) So, what did my IF plan look like? My day started off at 7 a.m. where I began with a cup of black coffee. I drank a little bit of water, then proceeded to perform 30 minutes of cardio, being sure to continue to drink water during my cardio session as well as after. My first meal would be eaten at 2 p.m, and my last meal would be finished by 10 p.m. I made a liberal use of water throughout the day, as it is an extremely underrated "metabolic fat flusher." Drinking a lot of water during the day also helped keep me stay satiated until my p.m. meal. IF does some very positive things to the metabolism, including the following:

AFFECTING INSULIN

When we eat, insulin increases. When we fast, insulin is decreased dramatically. This lower level of insulin promotes fat burning.

AFFECTING GROWTH HORMONE

Growth hormone levels have been shown to explode during a fast, as much as 5-fold. Growth hormone is a hormone that can be key in both fat burning and muscle gain, which is exactly what we are looking for.

AFFECTING NOREPINEPHRINE

During fasting, norepinephrine is sent to the fat cells by the nervous system, causing the fat cells to break down body fat into free fatty acids that can be burned for energy.

My keys to success with IF were: eating as much during the 8-hour eating window as I did on my "regular" eating plan and continuing to eat the same foods that I regularly ate. I am by no means giving you an exhaustive explanation here of IF. Do your research on the various interpretations of intermittent fasting and use the one that is best for you. Give it a try. You will not be disappointed with the results!

> "I'm not sold on one diet philosophy. I'm sold on whatever will work for you."
> -Dave Tate

Chapter 53

HOW TO EAT FOR LEAN MUSCLE MASS GAINS

One must be careful to eat plenty of the foods that help acquire muscle mass and avoid foods that can hurt muscle gain efforts. A muscle gain plan will have plenty of nutrient dense food such as lean beef, lean pork, chicken, eggs, fish, milk, whey protein, legumes, nuts, brown rice, oats, and lots of water. Foods to be avoided include fast food meals, processed meals and snacks, and anything with an overabundance of saturated fats or sugar.

I often scramble to get out of the house in the morning, and a protein drink is often a convenient choice for my breakfast. I prefer whey protein over others, as recent studies have shown that whey protein is most effective in increasing muscular hypertrophy over other protein powder choices.

Muscle mass calorie requirements are based on the number of calories that your body burns per day. This number will vary from one individual to the other. Basically, you will need your body to be in a caloric surplus to build muscle. Science does not have a consensus on exactly how much the surplus should be. This part of the muscle mass building equation will take some experimentation on your part. Take into consideration that a professional bodybuilder makes eating pretty much a full-time job! Not saying you need to emulate 100% the way a professional bodybuilder eats, but it implies that if you want to gain muscle mass you must eat up!

A basic lean muscle mass eating program will include three meals per day including a snack between each meal. Figure out your meal and snack macronutrient totals to ensure that you get in 1 gram of protein per pound of desired bodyweight per day. This is a good guideline to follow when eating to increase muscle. Meal timing in relation to your weight training workouts are important as well. There is a metabolic window that will be open up to 45 minutes after your workout. Eating within this metabolic window is important for recovery and muscle gain.

Through my own experimentation, I have found that having a minimum serving of 40 grams of protein before retiring for bed has resulted in significant increases in lean body mass and strength. More importantly, recent research has been done on the subject and it appears to be a major breakthrough in protein timing and muscle gain.

One must be careful to avoid certain nutritional pitfalls in the quest to gain lean muscle mass. The big ones in this category are not eating enough calories, not eating enough carbohydrate, not getting enough rest and sleep, and the utilization of ineffective resistance training routines.

The following is an example of how I eat on a typical day to gain lean body mass:

HOW TO EAT FOR LEAN MUSCLE MASS GAINS

BREAKFAST:
I like to start the day with a whey protein drink along with a cup of oatmeal mixed with blueberries and cinnamon.

SNACK:
A bag of Quest protein chips with bottled water.

LUNCH:
Two chicken breasts with a cup of brown rice along with a mix of zucchini, squash, onions, and water.

SNACK:
Hard boiled eggs with walnuts or almonds and maybe some raw broccoli with some low-fat dip.

DINNER:
Two lean grilled pork chops, large sweet potato, green beans, water.

BEFORE BED SNACK:
40 grams of whey protein mixed with 1 cup of 1% milk, one whole wheat muffin.

I average a body weight of about 233 pounds depending on my activity level. Thus, this amount of food might be a bit too much for many of you. It is simply a guideline as to how I do it. You can scale my plan down to meet your current macronutrient needs. However, you will find these nutritional tips for gaining lean body mass very helpful if you put them in to play!

"Sell yourself short on nutrition and you're selling yourself short on maximizing your physique development."

-Ernie Taylor

Chapter 54

A MYTH ABOUT PROTEIN INTAKE

For years we have been led to believe that our bodies can only absorb 20-30 grams of protein per meal. We were taught to spread out this amount of protein over 6 meals so it can be absorbed and utilized properly. When you do the math on this, it only comes out to a daily total of about 180 grams of protein per day if you are taking in just 30 grams of protein 6 times per day. When you consider a general protein requirement of 1 gram per pound of body weight for growth and repair for bodybuilding/weight training, 180 grams of protein per day is just not enough for someone much over 180 lbs.

However, there is much evidence that we can absorb much more protein per meal than this. How do you explain individuals who are eating 1.5 grams of protein per pound of body weight being a big and ripped 220 lbs. or more? How does a man or woman on an intermittent fasting eating plan utilize 50 to 100 grams of protein per meal in 2 or 3 meals over an 8-hour period and have the best physical condition of their life?

Research in this area is rather unclear and inconclusive. There are studies that indicate that the most important factor of protein synthesis is daily protein intake. I personally take in about 40 grams of protein per meal, 6 times per day. I weigh 233 lbs, so I average a little more than 1 gram of protein per pound of body weight ingested daily. This has worked quite well. So, what is the takeaway? HIT YOUR DAILY PROTEIN GOAL for the day and don't be too hung up on how you get there.

As stated earlier, some hard training lifters go for 1.5 grams of protein per pound of body weight, but I think a 1 gram per pound ratio is easily enough. So, if you are 150 pounds, get in 150 grams of quality protein per day. If you achieve or slightly exceed this goal by eating 40 g of protein per meal 4 times per day, you will be doing fine! Just strive to reach your daily protein goals without agonizing too much about how you space out your protein intake.

"To eat is a necessity, but to eat intelligently is an art."
- La Rochefoucald

FINAL WORDS

It must be stated that the training philosophies in this book are not the final word on how to build the body. The same goes for what you have learned from this book about cardiovascular exercise and nutrition. As my father often told me, "There is more than one way to skin a cat." However, what has been presented to you in *Motivated and Fit* represents some of the most time-tested, real-world methods available to the drug-free and genetically typical individual. The information in this book is largely what I have used for nearly 4 decades as the foundation of my fitness lifestyle. These are the things that have worked for me over the course of my training lifetime. I am living proof that utilizing a well thought out, progressive fitness program can result in a body that will almost miraculously change how you look and feel.

However, there are no magic pills when it comes to attaining the body of your dreams. Consistency in your training, focused effort on a nutritional program, and having a tenacious mindset are required. You are now holding in your hands the keys to creating a positive, lifelong change in your mind and body. IT'S UP TO YOU to use these keys in order to open up your own doors to success.

And please remember that you will not be alone on your journey. I am accessible to various forms of social media to help you on your path to success. You can reach me through the following methods:

Instagram - @JoelLuckyFitness
YouTube - JoelLuckyFitness
Facebook - facebook.com/joelluckyfitness
Website: JoelLucky.com

Now, take massive action and...
Get MOTIVATED and FIT!

Printed in Great Britain
by Amazon